Paediatrics at a Glance

Companion website

This book has an accompanying website at:

www.ataglanceseries.com/paediatrics

Features:

- Interactive self-assessment case studies from the book
- List of online resources

Paediatrics at a Glance

Lawrence Miall

MBBS, BSc, MMedSc, MRCP, FRCPCH
Consultant in Neonatal Medicine and Honorary Senior Lecturer
Leeds Teaching Hospitals NHS Trust and University of Leeds
Leeds

Mary Rudolf

MBBS, BSc, DCH, FRCPCH, FAAP
Professor of Child Health and Consultant Paediatrician
University of Leeds and Leeds Community Health Care Trust
Leeds General Infirmary
Leeds

Dominic Smith

MBBS, MMedSc, MRCP, MRCPCH
Consultant Paediatrician
Department of Child Health
York Teaching Hospital and Hull York Medical School
York

Third Edition

⊕WILEY-BLACKWELL

A John Wiley & Sons, Ltd., Publication

This edition first published 2012 © 2012 by John Wiley & Sons, Ltd

Wiley-Blackwell is an imprint of John Wiley & Sons, formed by the merger of Wiley's global Scientific, Technical and Medical business with Blackwell Publishing.

Registered office: John Wiley & Sons, Ltd, The Atrium, Southern Gate, Chichester, West Sussex, PO19 8SQ, UK

Editorial offices: 9600 Garsington Road, Oxford, OX4 2DQ, UK
The Atrium, Southern Gate, Chichester, West Sussex, PO19 8SQ, UK
111 River Street, Hoboken, NJ 07030-5774, USA

For details of our global editorial offices, for customer services and for information about how to apply for permission to reuse the copyright material in this book please see our website at www.wiley.com/wiley-blackwell.

Library of Congress Cataloging-in-Publication Data
Miall, Lawrence.
  Paediatrics at a glance / Lawrence Miall, Mary Rudolf, Dominic Smith. – 3rd ed.
      p. ; cm. – (At a glance)
  Includes bibliographical references and index.
  ISBN 978-0-470-65452-1 (pbk. : alk. paper)
  I. Rudolf, Mary. II. Smith, Dominic, 1970– III. Title. IV. Series: At a glance series (Oxford, England)
  [DNLM: 1. Pediatrics–methods–Handbooks. WS 39]
  618.92–dc23
                                              2011042664

A catalogue record for this book is available from the British Library.

Wiley also publishes its books in a variety of electronic formats. Some content that appears in print may not be available in electronic books.

Set in 9/11.5 pt Times by Toppan Best-set Premedia Limited
Printed and bound in Malaysia by Vivar Printing Sdn Bhd

1   2012

Contents

Companion website: www.ataglanceseries.comlpaediatrics

Preface to the third edition

"'What is the use of a book,' thought Alice, 'without pictures or conversations?'" Lewis Carroll, *Alice in Wonderland*

Paediatric medicine requires an understanding of developing anatomy, physiology and psychology as well as a holistic family-orientated approach. There are a wide range of professional challenges: from the technical aspects of intensive care to the ethical and sociological questions relating to issues of autonomy, independence and children's rights. The paediatric environment is very different to the world of adult medicine. This can all be daunting to those who are new to the specialty but developing the skills and confidence in successfully managing these challenges can enable professionals to make significant differences to the lives of children and families. This makes paediatric medicine amongst the most rewarding of all the medical specialties.

In preparing the third edition we have updated the text to reflect changes in understanding of childhood illness over the last 5 years. The new edition includes advances in genetics, screening and therapy of childhood illness. Topics have been updated to incorporate UK national guidelines on childhood urinary tract infection, constipation, fever, allergy, diabetes and meningitis.

Children have complex needs which require medical staff to work together with other professionals in child health, psychology, education and social care. There is increasing recognition of the need for all health professionals to have a good understanding of their role in safeguarding vulnerable people. New chapters have been added to expand on psychological issues and ethics in child health. There is greater detail on the recognition, investigation and management of child abuse.

We hope that this edition will continue to educate and inspire students and trainees in taking the first steps towards an understanding of children, their illnesses, their resilience in the face of adversity and amazing capacity for recovery. It is a book with many pictures to aid the introduction and revision of the key topics. We hope this will help as students begin their all-important conversations with young patients.

Lawrence Miall
Mary Rudolf
Dominic Smith

Preface to the first edition

He knew the cause of every maladye,
Were it of hoot or cold or moiste or drye,
And where engendred and of what humour:
He was a verray parfit praktisour.
> Geoffrey Chaucer c.1340–1400
> *A Doctor of Medicine, From Prologue to The Canterbury Tales*

Chaucer outlined with some clarity the qualities that a doctor of medicine requires, and emphasized that knowledge about the causes of maladies was required to come to competent diagnosis. We have structured *Paediatrics at a Glance* around children's common symptoms and maladies, and the likely causes for them. We have also attempted to distil for the student not only the knowledge base they require but in addition the competencies they must acquire in order to become 'verray parfit praktisours' when working with children and their parents.

The world has changed since Chaucer's time, and it is now widely acknowledged that the medical curriculum suffers from 'information overload'. We have made great efforts to adhere to the General Medical Council's recommendations in *Tomorrow's Doctors*, and have only included the core knowledge that we consider is required by doctors in training. We have in addition placed great emphasis on the evaluation of the child as he or she presents.

The focus of the book is similar to its parent book *Paediatrics and Child Health*. In both we have attempted to provide a working approach to paediatric problems and child health as they present in primary, community and secondary care. We have now taken the familiar *At a Glance* format and have visually presented each common symptom and led the student through the causes and key components of the evaluation so that a competent diagnosis can be made. Chapters are also devoted to providing the reader with an understanding of children's development and their place in society with additional chapters on nutrition, childcare, education and community services.

Although this book is principally intended for medical students, it may well provide appropriate reading for nurses and other allied professionals who would like to deepen their understanding of children and paediatric management. It is particularly likely to appeal to those who take a visual approach to learning.

Hippocrates wrote in his *Aphorisms for Physicians*, 'Life is short, science is long, opportunity is elusive, experience is dangerous, judgement is difficult'. We have produced this concise volume in the hope that it will help students cope with these hurdles to medical training, and facilitate the development of clinical acumen in their work with children.

Lawrence Miall
Mary Rudolf
Malcolm Levene

Acknowledgements

Various figures are taken from: Rudolf, M.C.J. & Levene, M.I. (2006) *Paediatrics and Child Health*, 2nd edn. Blackwell Publishing Ltd., Oxford.

4 Growth and puberty
Page 21—Child growth foundation.
Page 23—Heffner, L.J. (2010) Chapter 12, *The Reproductive System at a Glance*, 3rd edition, Blackwell Publishing Ltd., Oxford.

5 Understanding investigations
Page 27—Figure 5.3: Courtesy of Dr Sue Picton.

19 Congenital heart disease
Page 56—British Heart Foundation.

50 Rashes—types of skin lesions
Page 110, Papule: courtesy of Dr Katherine Thompson.
Page 110, Macule and Wheal: Courtesy of Mollie Miall.

51 Rashes—newborn, infancy and congenital skin disorders
Page 111, Cafe au Lait spots: Harper, J., Oranje, A. & Prose, N. S. (2006) Figure 19.13.2, p.1471. *Textbook of Pediatric Dermatology*, 2nd edition, Blackwell Publishing, Ltd., Oxford.

Page 111, Depigmentation: Harper, J., Oranje, A. & Prose, N. S. (2006) Figure 19.14.10, p.1496. *Textbook of Pediatric Dermatology*, 2nd edition, Blackwell Publishing, Ltd., Oxford.
Page 112, Erythema toxicum neonatorum: Harper, J., Oranje, A. & Prose, N. S. (2006) Figure 1.4.7, p.60. *Textbook of Pediatric Dermatology*, 2nd edition, Blackwell Publishing, Ltd., Oxford.

52 Rashes—infections and infestations
Page 113, Chickenpox: Harper, J., Oranje, A. & Prose, N. S. (2006) Figure 5.3.6, p.404. *Textbook of Pediatric Dermatology*, 2nd edition, Blackwell Publishing, Ltd., Oxford.
Page 113, Glass test: Courtesy of The Meningitis Trust.

56 The collapsed child
Page 123, Paediatric Life Support Algorithm and paediatric choking treatment algorithm: Reproduced with the kind permission of the Resuscitation Council (UK).

With thanks to our colleagues Dr Fiona Campbell, Dr Adam Glaser, Dr John Puntis, Dr Keith Brownlee, Dr Fauzia Khan, Dr Colin Ferrie, Dr Joanna Thomas and Dr Helen Bedford for their constructive reviews of various chapters.

Key to symbols used in the text

We have highlighted some likely and serious diagnoses at various points in the text, indicated by the following flag symbols for quick reference:

▻ Likely diagnosis
▶ Serious diagnosis

Abbreviations

AABR	automated auditory brainstem response	EEG	electroencephalogram
ACTH	adrenocorticotrophic hormone	ENT	ear, nose and throat
ADD	attention deficit disorder	ESR	erythrocyte sedimentation rate
ADH	antidiuretic hormone	FBC	full blood count
ADPKD	autosomal dominant polycystic kidney disease	FDP	fibrin degradation product
AFP	alpha-fetoprotein	FSGS	focal segment glomerulosclerosis
AIDS	acquired immunodeficiency syndrome	FTT	failure to thrive
ALL	acute lymphoblastic leukaemia	G6PD	glucose 6-phosphate dehydrogenase
ALT	alanine transaminase	GCS	Glasgow Coma Scale
ALTE	acute life-threatening event	GH	growth hormone
AML	acute myeloid leukaemia	GI	gastrointestinal
ANA	antinuclear antibody	GOR	gastro-oesophageal reflux
APTT	activated partial thromboplastin time	GP	general practitioner
ARPKD	autosomal recessive polycystic kidney disease	GTT	glucose tolerance test
ASD	atrial septal defect	HAART	highly active antiretroviral therapy
ASOT	antistreptolysin O titre	Hb	haemoglobin
AVPU	alert, voice, pain, unresponsive	HbF	fetal haemoglobin
AVSD	atrioventricular septal defect	HbS	sickle cell haemoglobin
AXR	abdominal radiograph	HIE	hypoxic-ischaemic encephalopathy
AZT	zidovudine (azidothymidine)	HIV	human immunodeficiency virus
BCG	bacille Calmette–Guérin	HPLC	high-performance liquid chromatography
BMI	body mass index	HSP	Henoch–Schönlein purpura
BP	blood pressure	HSV	herpes simplex virus
BSER	brainstem evoked responses	HUS	haemolytic uraemic syndrome
CDH	congenital dislocation of the hip	ICP	intracranial pressure
CF	cystic fibrosis	Ig	immunoglobulin
CFTR	cystic fibrosis transmembrane regulator	IM	intramuscular
CFU	colony-forming unit	INR	international normalized ratio
CHARGE	coloboma, heart defects, choanal atresia, retarded growth and development, genital hypoplasia, ear anomalies	IO	intraosseous
		IRT	immunoreactive trypsin
		ITP	idiopathic thrombocytopenic purpura
CHD	congenital heart disease	IUGR	intrauterine growth retardation
CMV	cytomegalovirus	IV	intravenous
CNS	central nervous system	IVC	inferior vena cava
CONI	care of the next infant	IVF	in-vitro fertilization
CPAP	continuous positive airway pressure	IVH	intraventricular haemorrhage
CPR	cardiopulmonary resuscitation	IVU	intravenous urogram
CRP	C-reactive protein	JCA	juvenile chronic arthritis
CRT	capillary refill time	LFT	liver function test
CSF	cerebrospinal fluid	LIP	lymphocytic interstitial pneumonitis
CSII	continuous subcutaneous insulin infusion	LMN	lower motor neuron
CT	computed tomography	LP	lumbar puncture
CXR	chest radiograph	Mag-3	radioisotope technetium ^{99m}Tc mertiatide
DDH	developmental dysplasia of the hip	MCAD	medium chain acyl-carnitine deficiency
DIC	disseminated intravascular coagulation	MCGN	minimal change glomerulonephritis
DIDMOAD	diabetes insipidus, diabetes mellitus, optic atrophy and deafness	MCH	mean cell haemoglobin
		MCUG	micturating cystourethrogram
DKA	diabetic ketoacidosis	MCV	mean cell volume
DM	diabetes mellitus	MDI	metered dose inhaler
DMD	Duchenne muscular dystrophy	MLD	mild learning difficulty
DMSA	dimercaptosuccinic acid	MMR	measles, mumps, rubella
DTPA	diethylenetriamine penta-acetate	MRI	magnetic resonance imaging
EBV	Epstein–Barr virus	MUAC	mid upper arm circumference
ECG	electrocardiogram	NEC	necrotizing enterocolitis
EDD	expected due date	NF	neurofibromatosis

NHL	non-Hodgkin's lymphoma
NICU	neonatal intensive care unit
NPA	nasopharyngeal aspirate
NSAID	non-steroidal anti-inflammatory drug
OAE	otoacoustic emissions
OFC	occipitofrontal circumference
ORS	oral rehydration solution
P_{CO2}	partial pressure of carbon dioxide
PCP	pneumocystis pneumonia
PCR	polymerase chain reaction
PCV	packed cell volume
PDA	patent ductus arteriosus
PEFR	peak expiratory flow rate
PKU	phenyketonuria
PNET	primitive neuroectodermal tumour
PR	per rectum
PT	prothrombin time
PTT	partial thromboplastin time
PUJ	pelviureteric junction
PUO	pyrexia of unknown origin
PVL	periventricular leucomalacia
RAST	radio-allergosorbent test
RBC	red blood cell
RDS	respiratory distress syndrome
RNIB	Royal National Institute for the Blind
ROP	retinopathy of prematurity
RSV	respiratory syncytial virus
SCBU	special care baby unit
SCID	severe combined immunodeficiency
SGA	small for gestational age
SIADH	syndrome of inappropriate antidiuretic hormone secretion
SIDS	sudden infant death syndrome
SLD	severe learning difficulty
SSPE	subacute sclerosing encephalitis
STD	sexually transmitted disease
SUDI	sudden unexpected death in infancy
T4	thyroxine
TAPVD	total anomalous pulmonary venous drainage
TB	tuberculosis
TGA	transposition of the great arteries
TNF	tumour necrosis factor
TORCH	toxoplasmosis, other (syphilis), rubella, cytomegalovirus, hepatitis, HIV
TS	tuberous sclerosis
TSH	thyroid stimulating hormone
tTG	tissue transglutaminase
U&E	urea and electrolytes
UMN	upper motor neuron
URTI	upper respiratory tract infection
UTI	urinary tract infection
UV	ultraviolet
VACTERL	vertebral anomalies, anal atresia, cardiac anomalies, tracheo-osophageal fistula, renal anomalies, limb defects
VER	visual evoked response
VKDB	vitamin K deficiency bleeding
VSD	ventricular septal defect
VUR	vesicoureteric reflux
WCC	white cell count

1 The paediatric consultation

The doctor–patient relationship

The consultation
- Introduce yourself to the child and parent
- Use emotional warmth and humour, and be patient
- Explain what will happen
- Use the child's name, engage the child, show interest in play
- Use a child-friendly environment
- Arrange the seating in a way which allows you to be alongside the parent in the discussion
- At the end, thank the child and explain what will happen next

Observations
- While taking the history start to observe the child and parent
- What is the interaction like?
- Consider child's development of movement, play and communication
- Are there any immediate signs of illness?
- Move on to measure height, weight and head circumference. Plot these on centile charts
- Examine for signs of acute illness
  - pulse
  - temperature
  - capillary refill time
  - blood pressure
  - respiratory rate
  - conscious level
- Assess for signs of pain
- Examine each system

Consent
- A child is legally defined as any individual below age 18 years
- An adult with parental responsibility can make a decision on behalf of the child up to age 18
- Children have rights as individuals
- Consent for examination and treatment is agreed with parent but the child should be involved in the discussion
- Older children who are competent to understand the significance of the issues may consent to examination and treatment without parents' knowledge but it is best practice to encourage the young person to involve their parents for support if possible

Communication skills in paediatrics

Paediatricians need to be happy with informality, enjoy humour and appreciate the unpredictability that children bring to consultations! Young children do not have a full understanding of the role of health professionals. Children will naturally be anxious and uncertain in an unfamiliar environment. They may not understand all of the language in the consultation but they quickly detect a sense of personal warmth, friendliness and relaxed mood in adults around them. It helps to have pictures, toys and videos to help children understand that the room is a good place for children.

In paediatrics the focus of the consultation changes with the age and understanding of the child. In a young baby the discussion is entirely with the carers (usually parents) who act as advocates for the child's needs. As children mature they need to be included in the discussion. It is important to understand the child's concerns and their right to be involved in decisions. Paediatricians need also to consider the concerns of the family and communicate sensitively with all family members.

Approaching the consultation

- Make friends with the child to gain their cooperation. Try to be confident and non-threatening. It may be best to examine an exposed part of the body first before undressing the child, or do a pretend examination on their teddy bear.
- Try to get down to the child's level—kneel on the floor or sit on the bed. Look at the child as you examine them. Use a style and

language that is appropriate to their age—'*I'm going to feel your tummy*' is good for a small child but not for an adolescent.

• Explain what you are going to do, but be careful of saying '*can I listen to your chest*' as they may refuse!

• Babies are best examined on a couch with the parent nearby; toddlers may need to be examined on the parent's lap.

• In order to perform a proper examination the child needs to be undressed, but this is often best done by the parent and only the region that is being examined needs to be undressed at any one time.

• Older children and adolescents should always be examined with a chaperone—usually a parent but, if the child prefers, a nurse. Allow as much privacy as possible when the child is undressing and dressing.

• Sometimes you may need to be opportunistic and perform whatever examination you can, when you can. Always leave unpleasant things until the end—for example; looking in the throat and ears can often cause distress.

• Hygiene is important, both for the patient and to prevent the spread of infection to other patients. Always wash your hands before and after each examination.

• Always sterilize or dispose of equipment that has been in contact with a patient, such as tongue depressors or auroscope tips.

History taking

The history often indicates the diagnosis before examination or investigations. The history can be taken from a parent, a carer or from the child. Record who gave the history and in what context. Use an independent interpreter if there are language difficulties.

Beginning the examination—observation

Much information can be gained by careful observation of the child. This starts while you are first talking to the parents.

• Signs of acute severe illness (need urgent intervention):
  – shock
  – severe respiratory distress
  – altered consciousness level
• Signs of pain or anxiety
• Growth and nutrition
• Features of syndromic disorders
• Developmental progress:
  – gross motor and fine motor movement
  – social interaction
  – speech and understanding
• Interaction with carers
• Hygiene and clothing
• Mood and behaviour

The examination of individual systems is discussed in detail on the following pages.

Presenting complaint	Record the main problems in the family's own words
History of presenting complaint	Try to get an exact chronology from the time the child was last completely well.
	Allow the family to describe events themselves; use questions to direct them and probe for specific information.
	Try to use open questions—'*tell me about the cough*' rather than '*is the cough worse in the mornings?*' Use direct questions to try to confirm or refute possible diagnoses.
Past medical history	In young children and infants this should start from the pregnancy, and include details of the delivery and neonatal period, including any feeding, growth or early development problems.
	Ask about all illnesses and hospital attendances, including accidents.
Developmental history	Milestones during infancy and school performance.
	Are there any areas of concern?
	Do the parents feel the child's development is comparable to their peer group?
	School performance—any academic or behavioural problems?
Immunizations	Review immunizations against national schedule.
	Are there any missed or extra vaccinations?
Drugs and allergies	What medication is the child taking? Include over the counter preparations.
	Does the child have any allergies to drugs or foods?
Systems enquiry	Ask a series of screening questions for symptoms within systems other than the presenting system
Family and social history	What is the family make-up and who lives at home?
	Draw a genogram with the family to discuss extended family history
	Consanguinity—having first-cousin parents increases the risk of genetic disorders
	Illnesses or developmental problems in the family
	Has there been any serious illness previously?
	Contact with infectious illness or foreign travel
Social history	Which school or nursery does the child attend?
	Parents' education background, jobs, physical and mental health
	Home environment—adults who smoke, housing problems, family stresses
Problem list	At the end of the history, prepare a clear problem list to guide further management

2 Systems examination

Respiratory system

Observation
- Is there respiratory distress?
  - nasal flaring, recession
  - use of accessory muscles
- Count the respiratory rate
- Is there wheeze, stridor or grunting?
- Is the child restless or drowsy?
- Is there cyanosis or pallor?
- Is there finger clubbing?
  - cystic fibrosis, bronchiectasis

Chest wall palpation
- Assess expansion
- Check trachea is central
- Feel apex beat
- Is there chest deformity?
  - Harrison's sulcus: asthma
  - barrel chest: air-trapping
  - pectus excavatum: usually isolated abnormality, can be associated with mitral valve prolapse or Marfan's syndrome
  - pectus carinatum (pigeon chest): idiopathic or associated with severe asthma
- May 'feel' crackles

Ear, nose and throat
- Examine eardrums using an auroscope
  - grey and shiny: normal
  - red and bulging: suggests otitis media
  - dull and retracted: chronic secretory otitis media (glue ear)
- Examine nostrils for inflammation, obstruction and polyps
- Examine pharynx using tongue depressor (leave this until last!)
  - Are the tonsils acutely inflamed (red ± pustules or ulcers) or chronically hypertrophied (enlarged but not red)
- Feel for cervical lymphadenopathy

Auscultation
- Use an appropriately sized stethoscope!
- Listen in all areas for air entry, breath sounds and added sounds
- Absent breath sounds in one area suggests pleural effusion, pneumothorax or dense consolidation
- With consolidation (e.g. pneumonia) there is often bronchial breathing with crackles heard just above the area of consolidation
- In asthma and bronchiolitis expiratory wheeze is heard throughout the lung fields
- In young children upper airway sounds are often transmitted over the whole chest. Asking the child to cough may clear them

Percussion note

Resonant	Normal
Hyper-resonant	Pneumothorax or air-trapping
Dull	Consolidation (or normal liver in right lower zone)
Stony dull	Pleural effusions

Age	Respiratory rate at rest (breaths/min)
<1	30–40
1–2	25–35
2–5	25–30
5–12	20–25
>12	15–20

KEY QUESTIONS FROM THE HISTORY

Breathlessness
- Consider the severity of breathing problems with activities
- Poor weight gain in infancy (a sign of respiratory distress)

Cough
- Chronology—any link to time of day/activity/environment
- Nature of cough: dry (viral), loose (productive), barking (croup), paradoxical (forced repetitive cough with difficult inspiration, seen in whooping cough)

Feeding in infancy
- Choking (gastro-oesophageal reflux)
- Symptoms with introduction of formula milk (cow's milk protein allergy)

Fever

Noisy breathing
- Noise in expiration (wheeze = lower airway obstruction)
- Noise in inspiration (stridor = upper airway obstruction)

Cough, wheeze or stridor in a young child
- If sudden onset, is there a history of inhaled foreign body or choking?

Ear, nose and throat
- Child pulling at their ears (middle ear infection)
- Difficulty in swallowing (tonsillitis or epiglottitis)
- Offensive odour breath (bacterial infection)
- Nasal secretions, bleeding

Family history
- Family history of respiratory problems (asthma, cystic fibrosis)
- Asthma, eczema, hay fever in close relative (atopy)
- Any smokers or pet animals in household?
- Travel to area of high tuberculosis prevalence, or contact with infected relative?

Cardiovascular system

Observation
- Is there central cyanosis? Peripheral cyanosis can be normal in young babies and those with cold peripheries
- If the child is breathless, pale or sweating this may indicate heart failure
- Is there finger clubbing? —cyanotic heart disease
- Is there failure to thrive? —suggests heart failure

Palpation
- Feel apex beat (position and character), reflects left ventricular function
- Feel for right ventricular heave over sternum (pulmonary hypertension)
- Feel for thrills (palpable murmurs)
- Hepatomegaly suggests heart failure. Peripheral oedema and raised JVP are rarely seen in children

Auscultation
- On the basis of the child's age, pulse, colour and signs of failure try to think what heart lesion may be likely, then confirm this by auscultation
- Listen for murmurs over the valve areas and the back (see p. 00). Diastolic murmurs are always pathological
- Listen to the heart sounds: are they normal, increased (pulmonary hypertension), fixed and split (ASD) or are there added sounds (gallop rhythm in heart failure or ejection click in aortic stenosis)?

Systolic murmur

Age	Systolic BP (mmHg)
<1	70–90
1–2	80–95
2–5	80–100
5–12	90–110
>12	100–120

Circulation
- Measure blood pressure with age-appropriate cuff, which should cover 2/3 of the upper arm
- Check capillary refill time (CRT) by pressing on the skin for 5 seconds—the time taken for the blanching to fade is the CRT. Normal is ≤2 s. A prolonged CRT >2 s may be a sign of shock. If the child is in a cold room peripheral CRT may be delayed, so always check centrally (e.g. over the sternum)

Pulse
- Rate: fast, slow or normal?

Age (years)	Normal pulse (beats/min)
<1	110–160
2–5	95–140
5–12	80–120
>12	60–100

- Rhythm: regular or irregular? Occasional ventricular ectopic beats are normal in children
- Volume: full or thready (shock)
- Character: collapsing pulse is most commonly due to patent arterial duct. Slow rising pulse suggests left ventricular outflow tract obstruction
- Always check femoral pulses in infants—coarctation of the aorta leads to reduced or delayed femoral pulses

KEY QUESTIONS FROM THE HISTORY

Medical condition associated with cardiovascular problems
- Genetic syndromes involving structural heart defects (e.g. Down's, Turner's, Marfan's syndromes)
- Renal problems (hypertension)
- Chemotherapy (some drugs cardiotoxic)

Breathlessness
- Breathing difficulties without signs of acute infection (consider cardiac disease)

Exercise
- Exercise limited by shortness of breath, palpitations or chest pain
- Competitive sports—rarely these may need to be limited with some cardiac defects

Colour change
- Cyanosis—central (tongue) or peripheral (hands and feet)
- Pale and sweaty, poor perfusion (sign of cardiac failure or an arrhythmia)

Growth
- Feeding problems in babies (breathlessness impairs feeding)
- Poor weight gain on growth chart

Syncope
- Unexplained collapse or fainting
- Collapse linked with exercise
- Palpitations
- Ask the parents to demonstrate rate/rhythm by tapping with their hand

Murmurs
- Previously noted heart murmur (physiological flow murmurs sometimes audible only at times of illness or after exercise)

Family history
- Family history of congenital heart disease
- Sudden death in early adulthood (congenital cardiomyopathy)

Abdominal system and nutritional status

Observation
- Make sure the child is relaxed
  - small children can be examined on a parent's lap, older children should lie on bed or couch
- Assess nutritional status
  - body mass index or mid-upper arm circumference
- Jaundice—yellow colour at skin and sclerae
- Pale if anaemic, most noticeable at palmar creases and conjunctivae
- Abdominal distension or oedema
- Wasting of buttocks (coeliac disease)

Palpation
- Check whether there is any pain before palpating
- Examiner should warm hands and get down to child's level
- Palpate 4 quadrants gently, check for tenderness
- Deeper palpation for organomegaly spleen, liver, kidneys
- Feel for any other masses, any palpable faecal loading in colon

Genitalia and anus
- Intimate examination should not be performed without senior staff supervision and chaperone
- Examine boys for hypospadias, undescended testes, hydrocoele, hernia

Percussion
- Shifting dullness with ascites
- Tympanic percussion with gaseous distension

Rectal examination
- This is very rarely indicated, but examine the anus for fissures or trauma

Auscultation
- Increased bowel sounds in obstruction
- Reduced in ileus

KEY QUESTIONS FROM THE HISTORY

Nutrition
- Infant feeding pattern—duration of breast-feeding
- Note any breast-feeding problems
- Is there a key professional to give support to breast-feeding?
- If formula milk fed, review type and volume (note: 1 fluid ounce = 28 mL)
- Review intake—typical infant intake is 100–150 mL/kg in 24 hours
- Age at weaning on to semi-solids, any choking problems, foods taken
- Detail what the child eats in a typical day
- Review calorie intake and nutritional balance
- Level of appetite, any difficult feeding behaviours
- Pattern of weight gain
- Review the parent-held health record (UK Red Book) growth pattern

Vomiting
- Vomiting frequency, colour
- Green vomit in infancy suggests bile (gastrointestinal obstruction)
- Posseting (small vomits of milk in mouth) in infancy suggests gastro-oesophageal reflux
- Blood in vomit in infancy suggests maternal blood swallowed with breast-feeding

- Blood in vomit in older children suggests oesophageal bleeding due to vomiting

Bowel habit
- Faeces—frequency, consistency, colour, any mucus, blood, greasy faeces
- Diarrhoea—frequency, consistency, urgency, blood, link with diet
- In newborn, meconium should be passed in first 24 hours after birth
- Age of potty training (child develops awareness and can control bowel movement to use potty)
- Constipation—straining, pain, reduced frequency, hard faeces
- Soiling of faeces in underwear (seen with overflow in constipation)
- Encopresis (behavioural problem of passing faeces in inappropriate place)

Pain
- Abdominal pain—site, radiation, chronology, nature, exacerbating and relieving factors

Family history
- Family history of liver, kidney, bowel disease

Genito-urinary symptoms
- Urinary frequency, dysuria, haematuria
- Enuresis (childhood urinary incontinence) by day and night
- Age at menarche, cycle frequency, regularity
- Menstrual bleeding flow, duration, pain symptoms

Neurological assessment

Observation

Conscious level

- AVPU scale = Alert/responds to voice/responds to pain/ unresponsive
- Glasgow coma scale

General observations

- Posture, movement and gait
- Limb deformity, contractures, hypertonicity
- Postural abnormalities in cerebral palsy:
  - diplegia, hemiplegia, quadriplegia
  - choreoathetoid movement
- Growth and head circumference
- Skin signs linked with neurological disorders (pigmentation, vascular birth marks)
- Dysmorphic features
- Equipment to aid neurological problems (e.g. hearing aid, limb splints, Pedro boots)

Tone

- Hypotonia suggests LMN lesion
- Spasticity suggests UMN lesion and is seen in cerebral palsy, especially in thigh adductors and calf muscles (may cause toe walking)

Power

- Describe in upper and lower limbs
- Describe whether movement is possible against resistance or against gravity

Peripheral exam

- Limbs —tone, power, coordination, muscle bulk, reflexes
- Gait (diplegia, hemiplegia, ataxia)
- Examine shoes for signs of unequal wear
- Sensation

Cranial nerves

- Examine as in adults
- Drooping mouth or expressionless face may be a sign of myopathy (e.g. myotonic dystrophy)

Facial exam

- Cranial nerves
- Eye exam, pupil reactions and fundoscopy

Coordination

- Finger–nose test and heel–shin test, and observe gait
  - Very important if considering CNS tumours as cerebellar signs are common

Developmental exam

- Part of complete neurological exam in children
  See Chapter 3

Reflexes

- Assess at knee, ankle, biceps, triceps and supinator tendons
- Clonus may be seen in UMN lesions
- Plantar reflex is upwards until 8 months of age, then downwards

---

KEY QUESTIONS FROM THE HISTORY

- Problems during pregnancy or neonatal period
- Review development:
  - loss of developmental milestone skills (regression, a sign of serious problems)
  - pattern of delay—global or limited (e.g. isolated speech and language delay)
- Headache symptoms
- Early morning vomiting (raised intracranial pressure)
- Involuntary movement, convulsion, unexplained collapse, altered consciousness level
- Sensory symptoms
- Urinary and faecal continence
- Hearing or vision problems, squint
- School performance
- Behaviour, mood, empathy, concentration
- Coordination, clumsiness, gait problems
- Function—how is the child limited by any neurological impairment?
- Home environment—any adaptations to assist care?
- Extra support received:
  - who assists with care of the child?
  - respite to parents
  - financial support to assist with care and mobility
- Family history of neurological problems:
  ○ epilepsy, blindness, deafness, learning difficulty, genetic disorder

The visual system

Observation of eyes

- Look at the iris, sclera and pupil
- Check pupils are equal and react to light, both directly and indirectly
- Look for red reflex to exclude cataract, especially in the newborn
- Look at reflection of light on the cornea—is it symmetrical or is one eye squinting? (see box opposite)
- Look at the inner epicanthic folds—if very prominent they may cause a pseudosquint

Normal symmetrical light reflex

Pseudosquint due to prominent inner epicanthic folds

Visual acuity

- Does the child fix and follow an object through 180 degrees?
- Can they see small objects (e.g. hundreds and thousands, small rolling Stycar balls)
- Older children can perform a modified Snellen chart with objects

Left convergent squint —note asymmetrical light reflex

Ocular movements and visual fields

- Test full range of movements, looking for paralytic muscle or nerve lesions
- Look for and describe any nystagmus
- Check visual fields by using a 'wiggling' finger

When the good eye is covered the squinting eye straightens (fixates)

Assessment of a squint

- Any squint in an infant beyond the age of 6 weeks needs referral to an ophthalmologist. A squinting eye that is left untreated may cause amblyopia (cortical blindness) on that side
- Some 'latent' squints are present only when the child is tired; the history is important
- Check the corneal light reflex at different angles of gaze
- Check ocular movements—is there a fixed angle between the eyes or a paralytic squint, where the squint increases with eye movement?
- Check visual acuity
- Perform fundoscopy and red reflex
- Perform the **cover test** by asking the child to fix on an object. Cover the 'good' eye and watch the squinting eye flick to fix on the object. Latent squints may also become apparent when that eye is covered
- Divergent squints are usually more pathological

Fundoscopy

- An essential but difficult skill—practise on every child you see!
- Look at the anterior chamber of the eye Cloudiness of the cornea suggests a cataract
- Examine the red reflex by looking through the ophthalmoscope held at a distance from the patient's eye. If the red reflex is absent this suggests cataract. A white reflex is suggestive of retinoblastoma
- Complete the examination by carefully examining the optic disc and retina

Neurological examination in infants

Young children cannot cooperate with a formal neurological examination so observation becomes more important: watch what the child is doing while you play with them

- How does the infant move spontaneously? Reduced movement suggests muscle weakness
- What position are they lying in? A severely hypotonic baby adopts a 'frog's leg' position (see below)
- Palpate anterior fontanelle to assess intracranial pressure and check head circumference
- Assess tone by posture and handling: a very floppy hypotonic baby tends to slip through your hands like a rag doll. Put your hand under the abdomen and lift the baby up in the ventral position: a hypotonic infant will droop over your hand. Pull the baby to sit by holding the baby's arms: observe the degree of head lag. Hypertonia is suggested by resistance to passive extension of the limbs and by scissoring (crossing-over) of the lower limbs when the infant is lifted up (see below)

Moro reflex	Symmetrical abduction and then adduction of the arms when the baby's head is dropped back quickly into your hand (see below). Usually disappears by 4 months
Palmar grasp	Stroking the palm causes hand to grasp. Usually disappears by 3 months
Asymmetrical tonic neck reflex	When the head is turned to one side the baby extends the arm on that side and flexes the contralateral arm ('fencing posture', see below). Disappears by 6–7 months

Scissoring of the lower limbs

'Frog's leg' position

Moro reflex

Asymmetric tonic neck reflex

Musculoskeletal system

Individual joint problems are discussed In Chapters 43 and 44

Observation
- Growth
- Joint inflammation
  – swelling, redness, heat, pain
- Limp or other functional impairment
- Signs of diagnosis linked to musculoskeletal problems
  – neurological (e.g. cerebral palsy, spina bifida)
  – genetic (e.g. neurofibromatosis, Marfan's syndrome)
- Skin signs (e.g. Henoch-Schönlein purpura, dermatomyositis)
- Skeletal deformity (e.g. spinal scoliosis)
- Ligamentous hyperlaxity

Joint examination
- Compare 2 sides
- Palpate all joints for swelling (effusion) and heat
- Test range of movement for all joints
- Observe for any pain during movement
- Examine for hip stability in newborn
- Check lengths are equal

Range of movements
- Assess the limit of active movements, then move the child's limb to assess passive movements.
  Observe the face for signs of pain, and stop before this occurs
- Check all the large joints in flexion, extension, rotation, abduction and adduction
- It is particularly important to check that the hip joints fully abduct in newborns and in children with cerebral palsy in order to exclude hip dislocation (see Chapter 42)

Scoliosis
- Observe the child standing—is there any asymmetry?
- Ask the child to flex their spine to touch their toes—scoliosis causes chest asymmetry with this movement
- Scoliosis can be part of a syndromic diagnosis or develop spontaneously through childhood or adolescence

Gait analysis
- Some centres use video gait analysis to measure gait anomalies and response to treatment (e.g. following botulinum toxin injections to leg muscles to reduce hypertonicity in cerebral palsy)

KEY QUESTIONS FROM THE HISTORY

Newborn
- Risk factors for congenital hip dysplasia—female, breech, family history

Older children
- Inflammation—joint pain, swelling, heat, restricted movement
- Limitation to activities (sports, walking distance)

- Gait problems:
  – limp with pain, hemiplegia
  – waddling gait with diplegia, muscle weakness, congenital dislocation of the hip.
  – tip-toe walking—often behavioural but may also be a sign of diplegic cerebral palsy
- Fever or skin rash (autoimmune disorders, septic arthritis)

3 Development and developmental assessment

- Parents are usually concerned if development is delayed but may not be aware of normal milestones so development should be reviewed by a trained health professional at critical stages in preschool years and at other health contacts such as attendance for immunization
- Development is an important indicator of a child's wellbeing. Delay or abnormal development may have serious consequences for later life
- Development problems can be a strong indicator of significant condition such as genetic disorder, structural neuroanatomical malformation or inborn error of metabolism

Tips on performing a developmental assessment
- Young children will not often immediately cooperate so use early opportunities to observe them informally
- You may have to rely heavily on parental report but, whenever possible, verify this through observation and testing with the child
- It is hard to remember all the milestones, so make sure you learn the essential points for key ages.
- Present the tasks one at a time
- Correct for prematurity until the child is 2 years old
- Measure milestones against a validated score, e.g. schedule of growing skills
- Define any delay as global or specific to a limited number of developmental areas, e.g. isolated speech and language delay
- Repeat assessments over months to measure the rate of development of new skills

Be systematic and evaluate the four developmental areas in turn

GROSS MOTOR

FINE MOTOR

SPEECH AND LANGUAGE

SOCIAL SKILLS

and also VISION AND HEARING

Standing and walking

6 months
Stands with support

10 months
Pulls to standing and stands holding on

12 months
Stands, and walks with one hand held

15 months
Walks independently and stoops to pick up objects

Gross motor development

Prone position

Birth
Generally flexed posture

6 weeks
Pelvis flatter

4 months
Lifts head and shoulders with weight on forearms

6 months
Arms extended supporting chest off couch

Pull to sit

Birth
Complete head lag

6 weeks
Head control developing

4 months
No head lag

Sitting

6 weeks
Curved back, needs support from adult

6–7 months
Sits with self propping

9 months
Gets into sitting position alone

Fine motor development

Grasping and reaching

4 months
Holds a rattle and shakes purposefully

5 months
Reaches for object

6 months
Transfers object from hand to hand

7 months
Finger feeds

Building bricks

12 months
Gives bricks to examiner

15 months
Builds a tower of two cubes

18 months
Builds a tower of three to four cubes

Manipulation

5 months
Whole hand grasp

9 months
Immature pincer grasp

10 months
Points at bead

12 months
Mature pincer grasp

Pencil skills

18 months
Scribbles with a pencil

3 years
Draws a circle

4 years
Draws a cross

5 years
Draws a triangle

Speech and language development

Speech

3 months
Vocalizes
ooh, aah

8 months
Double babble
dada baba mama

12 months
Two or three words with meaning
Mummy

3 years
Full sentences, talks incessantly
Teddy goes to sleep
Teddy's tired
Good night Teddy

18 months
10 words
Teddy Ta Bottle
Bed Dog No
Daddy Bikky

24 months
Linking two words
Daddy gone

Social development

6 weeks
Smiles responsively

16 weeks
Laughing out loud

7 months
Stranger anxiety

9 months
Peek a boo, waves bye bye

15 months
Drinks from a cup

18 months
Spoon-feeding self

About 2½ years (very variable)
Toilet trained by day

3 years
Dresses self (except buttons)

An assessment of developmental progress is important at every clinical encounter with children. It is important to understand the normal progression of development in the early years and to develop skills in examination to assess development in babies and children of different ages.

Milestones

It is hard to remember all the milestones, so learn the essential ones given in the table.

Milestones that are essential to remember

Age	Milestone
4–6 weeks	Fixes to faces with eyes
	Smiles responsively
6–7 months	Sits up unsupported
9 months	Gets to a sitting position
10 months	Pincer grasp
	Waves bye-bye
12 months	Walks unsupported
	Two or three words with meaning
18 months	Feeds self with spoon
	Points to things
	Tower of 3–4 cubes
	Throws a ball without falling
24 months	Sentences of 2–3 words
	Running
	Kicks a ball

Developmental warning signs

There is a wide variation in the age at which milestones are met. Key warning signs of significant developmental problems are listed in the table.

Key developmental warning signs

Age	Warning sign
At any age	Maternal concern
	Regression in previously acquired skills
10 weeks	No smiling
6 months	Persistent primitive reflexes
	Persistent squint
	Hand preference
	Little interest in people, toys, noises
10–12 months	No sitting
	No double-syllable babble
	No pincer grasp
	Not chewing
18 months	Not walking independently
	Less than 6 words
	Persistent mouthing and drooling
2½ years	No 2–3 word sentences
	Not responding to 1-word commands
	Not turning single pages
	No symbolic play
4 years	Unintelligible speech

KEY POINTS

- Develop your examination skills by assessing the development of any preschool child you encounter.
- Correct for prematurity, but remember premature babies are at increased risk of developmental delay.
- Early recognition aids diagnosis of underlying disorders and allows the child to access targeted developmental therapy.
- See Chapter 38 for causes of delayed development.

Growth and puberty

Growth

Accurate measurement of growth is a vital part of the assessment of children. In order to interpret a child's growth, measurements must be plotted on a growth chart. If there is concern about growth, the rate of growth must be assessed by measuring the child on two occasions at least 4–6 months apart.

Height
- Use a properly calibrated standing frame
- The child should be measured barefoot with knees straight and feet flat on the floor
- Stretch the child gently and read the measurement

Length
- The child should be measured lying down until 2 years of age
- Measuring the length of infants requires skill
- Use proper equipment and two people to hold the child

Weight
- Scales must be calibrated accurately
- Babies should be weighed naked (no nappy!)
- Older children should be weighed in underwear only

Head circumference
- Use flexible non-stretchable tape
- Obtain three successive measurements and take the largest to be the occipito frontal circumference (OFC)

GROWTH CHART

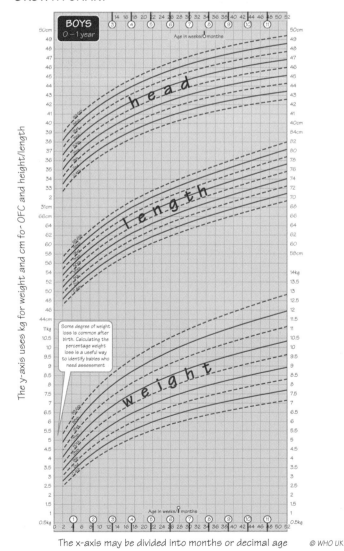

The x-axis may be divided into months or decimal age   © WHO UK

Plot on a growth chart

In the UK the UK-WHO charts are used for children aged 0–4 years and the UK 1990 charts for older children
- Nine equidistant centile lines are marked
- The weight centiles are splayed as the population is skewed towards being overweight
- The 50th centile is the median for the population
- A measurement on the 98th centile means only 2% of the population are taller or heavier than the child
- A measurement on the 2nd centile means that only 2% of the population are lighter or shorter than the child

Principles of plotting
- The child's measurement should be marked with a dot (not a cross or circle)
- Correct for prematurity up to the age of 1 year at least
- Height should follow one centile between 2 years and puberty
- Infants may normally cross centiles in the first year or two, but consider whether weight faltering or excess weight gain is a problem
- Infants may normally cross centiles in the first year or two, but consider whether failure to thrive is a problem (see Chapter 15)
- A child's final height is expected to fall midway between the parents' centile positions

Examples of growth charts

► Prematurity

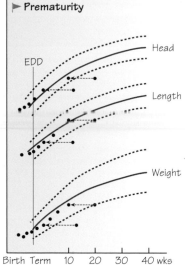

Birth Term 10 20 30 40 wks

Premature baby
- This child was born at 30 weeks and dicharged home at term. He is seen in clinic at 12 weeks (2 weeks CGA) and at 20 weeks (10 weeks CGA). Horizontal arrows show the correction for prematurity.

Coeliac disease

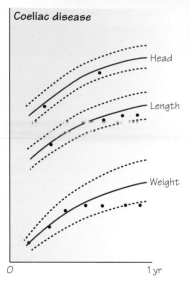

0   1 yr

Coeliac disease
- Note fall-off in weight at time of weaning when wheat was introduced
- The fall-off in length follows later

► Intrauterine growth retardation

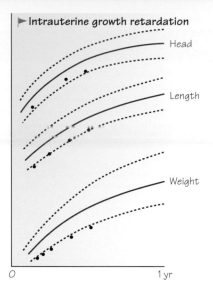

0   1 yr

Intrauterine growth retardation (IUGR)
- Low birthweight baby
- Many IUGR babies show catch-up but this baby clearly has not, and may have reduced growth potential
- The IUGR probably started early in pregnancy because head circumference and length are also affected

► Hydrocephalus

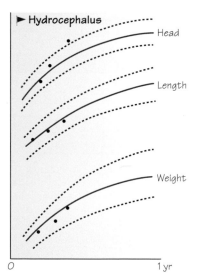

0   1 yr

Hydrocephalus
- The head circumference is crossing centile lines upwards
- A normal but large head would grow above but parallel to the centile lines

Turner's syndrome

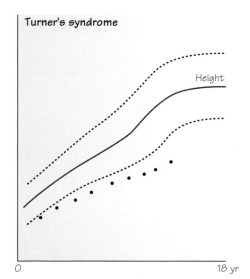

0   18 yr

Turner's syndrome
- There is poor growth from a young age
- Absence of pubertal growth spurt
- The child should have been referred for growth-promoting treatment when young

Growth hormone deficiency

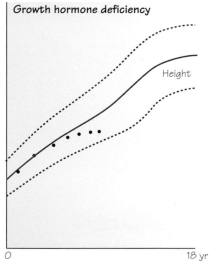

0   18 yr

Growth hormone deficiency
- Note the fall-off in height
- GH deficiency is rare
- It can be congenital, but as growth has plateaued at the age of 6 years, pituitary deficiency due to a brain tumour must be considered
- Acquired hypothyroidism has a similar growth pattern

Puberty

Puberty is evaluated by clinical examination of the genitalia, breasts and secondary sexual characteristics. The scale used is known as Tanner staging.

Boys

Genital development

Stage 1   Stage 2   Stage 3   Stage 4   Stage 5

Pubic hair growth

Stage 2   Stage 3   Stage 4   Stage 5

Girls

Breast development

Stage 1   Stage 2   Stage 3   Stage 4   Stage 5

Pubic hair growth

Stage 2   Stage 3   Stage 4   Stage 5

Principles of puberty

- The first signs of puberty are usually testicular enlargement in boys, and breast budding in girls.
- Puberty is precocious if it starts before the age of 8.5 years in girls and 9.5 years in boys.
- Puberty is delayed if onset is after 13 years in girls and 14 years in boys.
- A growth spurt occurs early in puberty for girls, but at the end of puberty for boys.
- Menarche occurs at the end of puberty. Delay is defined as no periods by 16 years of age.

Understanding investigations:
I Haematology

Investigations should only be requested to confirm a clinical diagnosis, or if indicated following a thorough history and examination. Sometimes they are performed to rule out more serious but less likely conditions. Blindly performing investigations as a 'fishing' exercise in the hope of throwing up an abnormality is usually counter-productive, often leading to increased anxiety and further investigations when unexpected results are obtained. These pages describe how to interpret some of the common investigations performed in paediatrics.

Haematology

Haemoglobin

Coombs test

- Detects the presence of IgG antibodies bound to the surface of RBCs leading to agglutination
- Useful in the diagnosis of immune mediated haemolytic anaemia (HA) such as autoimmune HA or haemolytic disease of the newborn

Blood film

This blood film shows erythrocytes, leucocytes and platelets. The blood film can be useful to identify abnormally shaped cells (e.g. spherocytosis) or primitive cells (e.g. lymphoblasts in leukaemia). It may show pale (hypochromatic) red cells in iron deficiency

Normal values

Haemoglobin	11 – 14 g/dL
Haematocrit	30 – 45%
White cell count	6 – 15 x 10⁹/L
Reticulocytes	0 – 2%
Platelets	150 – 450 x 10⁹/L
MCV	76 – 88 fL
MCH	24 – 30 pg
ESR	10 – 20 mm/h

White cell count $6 - 15 \times 10^9/L$, Platelets $150 - 450 \times 10^9/L$.

Mean cell volume (MCV)

- Measures the size of RBCs
- Microcytic anaemia (MCV <76 fL) is usually due to iron deficiency, thalassaemia trait or lead poisoning
- Macrocytosis may reflect folate deficiency

Mean cell haemoglobin (MCH)

- Reflects the amount of haemoglobin in each red cell. Is usually low (hypochromic) in iron deficiency

Flow diagram to show the investigation of anaemia

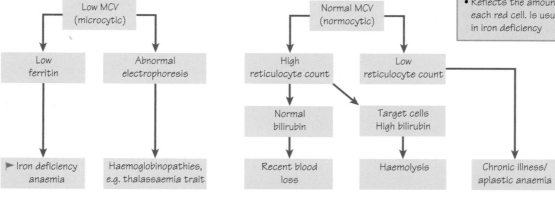

Platelets

- High platelet count usually reflects bleeding or inflammation (e.g. Kawasaki disease)
- Low platelet count is commonly seen with idiopathic thrombocytopenic purpura (ITP) when there is a risk of spontaneous bruising and bleeding. In the newborn it may be low due to maternal IgG-mediated immune thrombocytopenia
- Platelets may sometimes be functionally abnormal (e.g. von Willebrand disease, Glanzmann disease or Bernard–Soulier disease) which requires further investigation

Clotting

- Prothrombin time (PT) compared with a control is used to calculate the INR: normal is 1.0. Principally assesses extrinsic pathway. Prolonged in vitamin K deficiency, liver disease and disseminated intravascular coagulation (DIC)
- Activated partial thromboplastin time (APTT) reflects the intrinsic pathway. Prolonged in heparin excess, DIC and haemophilia A
- Fibrin degradation products (FDPs) are increased in DIC
- Bleeding time: literally the time a wound bleeds for. Prolonged in von Willebrand disease and thrombocytopenia
- Specific clotting factor assays are performed in the investigation of haemophilia and other bleeding disorders

White blood cells

- Leucocytosis usually reflects infection—neutrophilia and 'left shift' (i.e. immature neutrophils) implies bacterial infection. Lymphocytosis is more common in viral infections, atypical bacterial infection and whooping cough
- Neutropenia (neutrophils < 1.0 x 10⁹/L) can occur in severe infection or due to immunosuppression. There is a high risk of spontaneous infection
- ► Leukaemia: There is usually a very high (or occasionally low) WCC with blast cells seen. Bone marrow aspirate is required (see Chapter 49)

 Paediatrics at a Glance, Third Edition. Lawrence Miall, Mary Rudolf, Dominic Smith. © 2012 John Wiley & Sons, Ltd. Published 2012 by John Wiley & Sons, Ltd.

Interpretation of blood gases

The acidity of the blood is measured by pH. Ideally blood gases should be measured on an arterial sample, but in babies capillary samples are sometimes used, which makes the Po_2 unreliable. A high pH refers to an alkalosis and a low pH to an acidosis. The pH is a logarithmic scale, so a small change in pH can represent a large change in hydrogen ion concentration. Once the blood becomes profoundly acidotic (pH<7.0), normal cellular function becomes impossible. There are metabolic and respiratory causes of both acidosis and alkalosis (see below). The pattern of blood gas abnormality (particularly the pH and Pco_2) can be used to determine the type of abnormality.

Metabolic acidosis
- ▶Severe gastroenteritis
- Perinatal asphyxia (build-up of lactic acid)
- Shock
- ▶Diabetic ketoacidosis
- Inborn errors of metabolism
- Loss of bicarbonate (renal tubular acidosis)

Respiratory acidosis
- Respiratory failure and underventilation

Metabolic alkalosis
- Usually due to vomiting, e.g. pyloric stenosis

Respiratory alkalosis
- Hyperventilation (e.g. anxiety)
- Salicylate poisoning: causes initial hyperventilation and then metabolic acidosis due to acid load

$$CO_2 + H_2O \rightleftharpoons H_2CO_3 \rightleftharpoons H^+ + HCO_3^-$$

Control of acid–base balance

Gas exchange   Renal adaptation

Compensation can occur by the kidneys, which can vary the amount of bicarbonate excreted. A persistent respiratory acidosis due to chronic lung disease will lead to retention of bicarbonate ions to buffer the acid produced by CO_2 retention. Hence, a **compensated respiratory acidosis** will have a low–normal pH, a high Pco_2 and a very high bicarbonate level

Normal arterial blood gas values

pH	7.35 – 7.42
Pco_2	4.0 – 5.5 kPa
Po_2	11 – 14 kPa (children)
	8 – 10 kPa (neonatal period)
HCO_3^-	17 – 27 mmol/L

Determining the type of blood gas abnormality (N = normal)

	pH	Pco_2	Po_2	HCO_3^-
Metabolic acidosis	Low	N	N	Low
Respiratory acidosis	Low	High	N/low	N
Metabolic alkalosis	High	N	N	High
Respiratory alkalosis	High	Low	N/high	N
Compensated respiratory acidosis	N	High	N	High

Electrolytes and clinical chemistry

Normal ranges

Sodium	135 – 145 mmol/L
Potassium	3.5 – 5.0 mmol/L
Chloride	96 – 110 mmol/L
Bicarbonate	17 – 27 mmol/L
Creatinine	20 – 80 μmol/L
Urea	2.5 – 6.5 mmol/L
Glucose	3.0 – 6.0 mmol/L
Calcium	2.15 – 2.70 mmol/L

Characteristic patterns of serum electrolyte abnormality sometimes suggest particular diagnoses:
- **Pyloric stenosis:**
  There is often a metabolic alkalosis, a low chloride and low potassium concentration (due to repeated vomiting and loss of stomach acid) and a low sodium concentration
- ▶**Diabetic ketoacidosis:**
  There is a metabolic acidosis with a very low bicarbonate, a high potassium, high urea and creatinine and a very high glucose concentration
- ▶**Gastroenteritis:**
  Urea concentration is high, but the sodium may be either high or low depending on the sodium content of the diarrhoea, and on the type of rehydration fluid that has been administered

Causes of abnormal sodium balance

Alterations in sodium concentration usually reflect changes in the level of hydration (total body water content). Serum sodium concentration must be corrected slowly, as a sudden fall in sodium can cause fitting

Hypernatraemia (Na^+ >145 mmo/L)
- Dehydration – fluid deprivation or diarrhoea
- Excessive sodium intake
  - inappropriate formula feed preparation
  - deliberate salt poisoning (very rare)

Hyponatraemia (Na <135 mmol/L)
- Sodium loss
  - diarrhoea (especially if replacement fluids hypotonic)
  - renal loss (renal failure)
  - cystic fibrosis (loss in sweat)
- Water excess
  - excessive intravenous fluid administration
  - SIADH (inappropriate antidiuretic hormone secretion)

Potassium

- **Hyperkalaemia:** High potassium levels can cause serious cardiac arrhythmias and need to be controlled rapidly. Check for a wide QRS complex and peaked T waves on ECG. The danger is exacerbated by low serum calcium concentration. Treatment includes salbutamol infusion, insulin and dextrose infusion (to drive potassium into cells) and rectal calcium resonium
- **Causes of hyperkalaemia (>5.5 mmol/L):**
  - renal failure or sudden oliguria
  - massive haemolysis or tissue necrosis
  - congenital adrenal hyperplasia
  - arteIfact (if difficulty obtaining sample)
- **Hypokalaemia (<3.5 mmol/L):** A low potassium causes muscle weakness, ileus and lethargy
- **Causes of hypokalaemia:**
  - diarrhoea and vomiting
  - diuretic therapy
  - inadequate intake (e.g. starvation)

Calcium
- Hypocalcaemia is most commonly caused by vitamin D deficiency and if extreme can present with weakness, tetany, cardiac arrhythmias and convulsions. Congenital hypocalcaemia is caused by hypoparathyroidism in DiGeorge syndrome
- Hypercalcaemia is rare in childhood and needs careful investigation. Various types of hyperparathyroidism may be present. Congenital hypercalcaemia may be seen in Williams syndrome or subcutaneous fat necrosis

Understanding investigations: II   Radiology

Features to look for on a chest radiograph

Radiograph of right middle and upper lobe pneumonia

Lateral radiograph showing right upper and middle lobe pneumonia

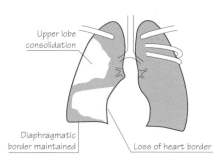

Upper lobe consolidation

Diaphragmatic border maintained

Loss of heart border

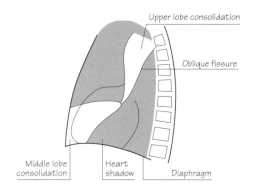

Upper lobe consolidation

Oblique fissure

Middle lobe consolidation

Heart shadow

Diaphragm

Chest radiography

As respiratory disorders are so common in paediatric practice, it is very important to be able to accurately interpret chest radiographs. If there is uncertainty the film should be discussed with an experienced radiologist.
• Identify the patient name, date and orientation (left and right).
• Check the penetration—the vertebrae should just be visible behind the heart shadow.
• Check that the alignment is central by looking at the head of the clavicles and the shape of the ribs on each side.
• Comment on any foreign objects such as central lines.
• Examine the bony structures, looking for fractures, asymmetry and abnormalities (e.g. hemivertebrae). Rib fractures are best seen by placing the radiograph on its side.
• Check both diaphragms and costophrenic angles are clear. The right diaphragm is higher than the left because of the liver. Check there is no air beneath the diaphragm (indicates intestinal perforation).
• Look at the cardiac outline. At its widest it should be less than half the width of the ribcage (cardiothoracic ratio <0.5), although in infants it can be wider due to the antero-posterior way the radiograph is taken.
• Look at the mediastinum—note that in infants the thymus gland can give a 'sail'-like shadow just above the heart.
• Check lung expansion—if there is air trapping the lung fields will cover more than nine ribs posteriorly, and the heart will look long and thin.

• Examine the lung fields looking for signs of consolidation, vascular markings, abnormal masses or foreign bodies.
• Check that the lung markings extend right to the edge of the lung—if not, consider a pneumothorax (dark) or a pleural effusion (opaque).
• Consolidation may be patchy or dense lobar consolidation. A lateral radiograph may be required to determine exactly which lobe is affected. A rule of thumb is that consolidation in the right middle lobe causes loss of the right heart border shadow and right lower lobe consolidation causes loss of the right diaphragmatic shadow.
• Always look at the area 'behind' the heart shadow for infection in the lingula. If the mediastinum is pulled towards an area of opacity, consider collapse rather than consolidation as the pathology.

MRI and CT scans

MRI (magnetic resonance imaging) uses radio waves and powerful electromagnetic fields to obtain detailed images, which can highlight different tissues. Images can be obtained in any plane. MRI has the great advantage of being free of ionizing radiation. The scanners are often claustrophobic and can be noisy, so young children may require a general anaesthetic.

MRI is very good at delineating tissues with high water content from those with high fat content. MRI can distinguish white matter from grey matter within the brain. It is the imaging of choice for the investigation of CNS abnormalities including spinal abnormalities. Increasingly it is being used for complex cardiac and joint imaging also. On a standard T2 weighted image, water (e.g. CSF or oedema) shows up white. On a T1-weighted image it shows dark.

CT scans

CT (computed tomography) scans also give axial images ('slices' through the body). They have the advantage of being significantly faster to perform than MRI scans, and the machines are quieter and less claustrophobic, so children can be scanned while awake. CT is predominantly in assessing traumatic brain injury and in imaging the lungs, and is particularly good at detecting acute haemorrhage. The disadvantage is there is a significant radiation exposure.

Figure 5.1 Axial T2-weighted MRI of an infant brain. The dark grey cortex is clearly distinguished from the deeper white matter (light grey). The lateral ventricles are filled with CSF. There are bilateral haemorrhages (black) within the subependyma (just outside the wall of the lateral ventricles—arrowed).

Figure 5.2 A sagittal T1-weighted image showing cerebral atrophy with increased CSF (dark) spaces around the brain. The corpus callosum, brainstem structures and cerebellum are clearly identified.

Figure 5.3 T1-weighted sagittal MRI scan showing a large optic glioma. Note the heterogeneous nature with solid and cystic areas. This tumour is characteristically associated with neurofibromatosis type 1.

Ultrasound

Ultrasound is an excellent investigation for children, since it is safe and non-invasive, and the ultrasound machine can often be brought to the patient's bedside. It is used extensively to obtain images of the abdominal and pelvic organs, and in newborn infants can be used to image the brain and the lower spinal cord. The examination is best performed in real time. Increasingly congenital abnormalities are detected antenatally by ultrasound examination, usually performed at 18–20 weeks gestation.

Figure 5.4 A large extradural haematoma secondary to a left parieto-occipital skull fracture. Note the midline shift and compression of the left lateral ventricle.

Figure 5.5 CT scan showing collapse and bronchiectasis in the right upper lobe.

Figure 5.6 Coronal ultrasound examination of the brain, performed in a preterm infant via the anterior fontanelle. The lateral ventricles are dilated and there is haemorrhage within right ventricle, with a large right sided parietal venous infarction.

Figure 5.7 Ultrasound scan of kidney showing gross hydronephrosis.

Understanding investigations: III   Microbiology

Different methods are available to detect infection. Some are non-specific, such as changes in blood inflammatory markers, and others give specific information about the exact infection. Proof of infection includes direct detection (e.g. microscopy, antigen detection, PCR), detection of an antibody response (serology) or culture of an organism from a normally sterile site.

Non-specific markers of infection

Leucocytosis	High white count (>15 × 10⁹/L) suggests inflammation or infection

Leucocytosis	High white count ($>15 \times 10^9/L$) suggests inflammation or infection High neutrophil count suggests bacterial infection Lymphocytosis is seen in viral or some atypical bacterial infection (e.g. whooping cough)
C-reactive protein (CRP)	An acute phase protein that normally rises within 24 hours of infection
Erythrocyte sedimentation rate (ESR)	A non-specific marker of inflammation. Rarely used

Blood culture

Culture of a pure growth of a bacterium (or occasionally a fungus) from blood is usually definitive proof of infection. However, if the culture is of several different organisms, or if low pathogenic bacteria normally found on the skin (such as coagulase-negative *Staphylococci*) are isolated then the result should be interpreted with caution. The way the blood sample is taken is crucial—the skin must be thoroughly cleaned with antiseptic and an aseptic technique used. Very small blood samples (<1 mL) reduce the chances of a positive culture. Blood cultures usually take 24–48 hours to show evidence of infection and so are usually used to confirm a clinical suspicion of infection retrospectively. Cultures will provide information about the sensitivity of the organism, which can be used to rationalize antibiotic therapy. Most modern blood culture systems are able to detect significant bacteraemia in children with a single medium, which is designed specifically for this purpose. Unusual results should always be discussed with a microbiologist.

Serological evidence of infection

Measurement of antibody response to specific infectious agents can be useful. This is important to check for prior immunity (for example in an at risk child vaccinated against hepatitis B) or to confirm prior infection (e.g. cytomegalovirus, CMV). IgG antibody tends to persist after infection whereas IgM antibody reflects recent infection. This can be important in the newborn period for distinguishing congenital infection (e.g. syphilis) from maternal infection, since IgG antibody readily crosses the placenta. Antibody responses to infection are often described as 'titres'. The titre is the reciprocal of the highest dilution of the patient's serum in which antibody was detected, e.g. a titre of 1024 means that antibody was detected in a 1:1024 dilution of serum. The higher the titre, the more antibody is present. The anti-streptolysin-O titre (ASOT) is sometimes used as a marker of streptococcal infection in rheumatic fever.

Direct detection methods

Molecular biology techniques can now identify certain organisms, such as viruses, that have traditionally been difficult to culture. These tests can either use immunofluorescence, e.g. to identify respiratory syncytial virus (RSV) in pharyngeal secretions in a child with bronchiolitis, or polymerase chain reaction (PCR) to amplify bacterial or viral DNA using specific primers. PCR methods are available for many important paediatric infectious agents, including herpes simplex virus (HSV), *Neisseria meningitidis* groups B and C, and HIV. They are particularly useful in confirming infection after antibiotics have already been given and in detecting viral CNS infection.

Lumbar puncture and CSF analysis

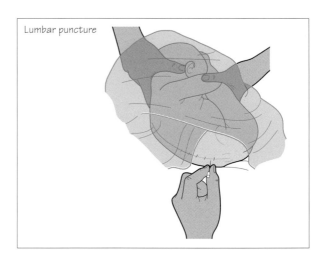

Lumbar puncture

Lumbar puncture is usually performed to diagnose or exclude meningitis. It should not be performed if there is evidence of raised intracranial pressure, if the child is haemodynamically unstable (e.g. septic shock) or if there is a low platelet count or coagulopathy. A fine spinal needle with a stylet is passed between the vertebral spines into the subdural space. A few drops of CSF are collected for microbiological examination and for analysis of protein and glucose concentrations. Examination of CSF includes microscopy and culture, and may also include other direct detection techniques (e.g. DNA detection with PCR). Normal CSF is usually 'crystal clear'. If it is cloudy, this suggests infection or bleeding. Fresh blood which clears usually indicates a traumatic tap, but a massive intracranial haemorrhage must be considered if the CSF remains bloodstained. Old blood gives a yellow 'xanthochromic' appearance. A manometer can be used to measure the CSF pressure, though this is not routinely performed.

Analysis of CSF

	Normal	Bacterial meningitis	Viral meningitis
Appearance	Crystal clear	Turbid, organisms seen	Clear
White cells	<5/mm^3	↑↑↑ (polymorphs)	↑ (lymphocytes)
Protein	0.15–0.4 g/L	↑↑	Normal
Glucose	>50% blood	↓	Normal

Although these are typical CSF findings for the organisms indicated, partially treated infection and infection with specific micro-organisms may result in alternative profiles. For example, meningitis caused by *Listeria monocytogenes* usually presents with a CSF lymphocytosis.

Urinalysis

Fresh urine should be collected into a sterile container from a midstream sample if possible. Urine bags applied over the genitalia may be used in infants, but often become contaminated with perineal bacteria.

• Observe the urine—is it cloudy (suggests infection) or clear?

• What is the colour?—pink or red suggests haematuria from the lower urinary tract; brown ('cola'-coloured) urine suggests renal haematuria or haemolytic disease (haemoglobinuria).

• Smell the urine for ketones and for the smell of infection. Unusual-smelling urine may suggest an inborn error of metabolism.

• Test the urine using commercial dipsticks. This may reveal:
  – protein—infection, renal damage or nephrotic syndrome
  – glucose—diabetes
  – ketones—diabetic ketoacidosis (DKA)
  – pus cells or nitrites—suggestive of infection

• These sticks are very sensitive to the presence of blood, and may detect haematuria even if the urine looks clear.

• Examine the urine under the microscope for white cells, red cells, casts and the presence of organisms. A sample should also be sent for culture. A pure growth of >10^5 colony-forming units of a single organism and >50 white cells/mm^3 confirms infection. Infection is extremely unlikely in the absence of pyuria.

Immunology

Immunological investigations may be needed to investigate a child with suspected immunodeficiency (severe, recurrent or unusual infections—see Chapter 22) or with an autoimmune disorder such as juvenile rheumatoid arthritis (see Chapter 22) or systemic lupus erythematosus or renal disease.

Basic immunological investigations include:

WBC	To ascertain the total number of white blood cells including neutrophils and lymphocytes (e.g. cyclical neutropenia)
T-cell subsets	To examine the number of CD4 and CD8 T-cells (e.g. HIV infection)
Immunoglobulins (IgG, IgM, IgA and IgE)	To investigate immunodeficiency with recurrent infections such as X-linked agammaglobulinaemia or severe combined immunodeficiency (SCID)
Functional antibodies	To detect specific IgG to confirm an adequate immune response to a trigger, such as *Haemophilus influenzae* immunization
Complement	May be low in certain immune-mediated kidney disorders (e.g. mesangiocapillary glomerulonephritis). Complement deficiency (e.g. C3 deficiency) is associated with recurrent infection of encapsulated organisms (e.g. *Neisseria meningitidis*)
Specific IgE antibodies	Used to investigate allergic disorders (see Chapter 54)
Specific antibody markers	IgA endomysial antibodies in coeliac disease (see Chapter 31)
	Antinuclear antibody (ANA) in juvenile idiopathic arthritis (see Chapter 44)

KEY POINTS

• Before ordering an investigation, consider how the result might alter the management.

• Try to focus investigations on the differential diagnosis based on clinical assessment.

• Sometimes investigations can be used to quickly rule out important or serious diagnoses (e.g. urine dipstix, CSF microscopy).

• Anyone who initiates a test request should ensure that the results are seen and dealt with appropriately.

6 The newborn baby

Gestation
- Full-term: born between 37 and 42 weeks' gestation
- Preterm: born before 37 completed weeks' gestation
- Post-term: born after 42 completed weeks

Birthweight
- Small for gestational age: birthweight <10th centile
- Very low birthweight: <1500 g
- Extremely low birthweight: <1000 g

The first breath
- Clamping the umbilical cord and response to cold stimulates the baby to take its first breath within a minute of birth
- Lung fluid is actively reabsorbed as well as being expelled during delivery
- Surfactant in the alveoli helps them to expand and fill with air
- Most babies can be dried and given straight to the mother. Occasionally, the onset of breathing may be delayed and the baby requires resuscitation

Vernix
- A white waxy substance that is often present, especially in preterm infants. Thought to provide insulation and lubrication

Breast-feeding
- A healthy baby can be put straight to the breast and will suckle soon after birth (see Chapter 10)

Mortality definitions
- Stillbirth: a baby (>24 weeks' gestation) who shows no signs of life after delivery (including no heart beat)
- Perinatal mortality rate: Stillbirths and deaths within the first week of life per 1000 births. Approximately 7/1000 in the UK
- Infant mortality rate: Number of deaths in the first year of life per 1000 live-born infants; approximately 5 per 1000

Umbilical cord
- Normally has two arteries and one vein
- After clamping it dries up and usually separates from the baby within the first week. It can be a site of infection

Resuscitation
- Usually, simple stimulation, drying and warming is sufficient but resuscitation may be needed in some babies
- Air or oxygen can be given by a pressure limiting device and mask and the baby placed under a warmer
- Intubation may sometimes be needed, especially if the baby has aspirated meconium or needs ongoing ventilation

Meconium
- Green–black stool passed by babies in the first days after birth
- Fresh meconium-stained liquor can be a sign of fetal distress but can be normal in full-term infants
- The asphyxiated gasping baby can aspirate meconium into the lungs, causing respiratory distress

Vitamin K
- Babies can sometimes be deficient in vitamin K, leading to severe bleeding disorders
- Vitamin K is routinely offered to all babies, either orally or by intramuscular injection. Breast-fed babies require three oral doses as breast milk contains less vitamin K than formula milks

The Apgar score

Score	0	1	2
Heart rate	Absent	<100	>100
Respiration	Absent	Irregular	Strong cry
Tone	Limp	Some flexion	Good flexion
Reflex to suction	None	Grimace	Cough or sneeze
Colour	White	Blue periphery	Pink

- The Apgar score is often used to describe the infant's condition at birth
- The score (0–10) is recorded at 1 min and 5 min of life
- A normal score at 1 min is 7–10
- Babies with a score of 0–3 at 1 min require rapid resuscitation or they will die

The normal newborn

The vast majority of babies are born at term, in good condition and do not require any medical involvement. Most babies in the UK are born in hospital, where a paediatrician is usually available to attend 'high risk' deliveries where it may be anticipated that resuscitation will be required. A healthy newborn term infant cries soon after birth, and is pink with good muscle tone, a normal heart rate and regular respiration. Once the cord has been clamped and cut, the baby can be dried and given straight to the mother for skin-to-skin contact and to establish breast-feeding. Newborn babies, especially if they are premature, are covered in a waxy material called vernix. Post-term infants may have very dry, cracked skin. Babies pass a green–black stool called meconium which changes to a normal yellow–brown stool after a few days.

It is recommended that infants are given vitamin K at birth to prevent potentially catastrophic bleeding. Newborn infants are routinely examined within the first few days to exclude congenital abnormalities (see Chapter 7) and have blood taken from a heel-prick around day 5 to screen for hypothyroidism and metabolic disorders (see Chapter 8).

►Asphyxia and resuscitation

The perinatal mortality rate (currently 7 per 1000) has halved in the UK over the last 20 years, largely due to improvements in obstetric care. The reduction in neonatal mortality rate (now less than 3 per 1000 live births) is due to improvements in the management of babies with complex congenital abnormalities and to improved care of preterm infants. Some babies still require immediate resuscitation after birth, and personnel attending deliveries must be trained in effective and rapid resuscitation. The need for resuscitation can often be anticipated and a paediatrician should be in attendance. Such situations include:

• Prematurity
• Fetal distress
• Thick meconium staining of the liquor
• Emergency caesarean section
• Instrumental delivery
• Known congenital abnormality
• Multiple births.

The condition of the infant after birth is described by the Apgar score (see opposite). Each of five parameters is scored from 0 to 2. A total Apgar score of 7–10 at 1 min of age is normal. A score of 4–6 is a moderately ill baby and 0–3 represents a severely compromised infant who may die without urgent resuscitation. Such babies will often require intubation and may require cardiac massage. In the most depressed babies IV drugs such as adrenaline (epinephrine) and bicarbonate may be necessary to re-establish cardiac output. The outcome for these infants may be poor.

Some infants in poor condition at birth may have suffered a hypoxic or ischaemic insult during pregnancy or labour. A healthy fetus can withstand brief physiological hypoxia, but an already compromised fetus may become exhausted and decompensate with build-up of lactic acid. These infants may develop irreversible organ damage, in particular to the brain. Umbilical cord blood gas samples should be assessed. Evidence of severe asphyxia includes a cord blood pH <7.0, Apgar score of <5 at 10 min, a delay in spontaneous respiration beyond 10 min and development of a characteristic hypoxic-ischaemic encephalopathy (HIE) with abnormal neurological signs including convulsions. Death or severe handicap occurs in more than 75% of the most severely asphyxiated term infants. Therapeutic hypothermia (cooling to 33 °C) for 72 hours may prevent secondary neuronal damage following moderate to severe asphyxia. However, for normal, well babies it is important to prevent hypothermia by careful drying and early skin-to-skin contact after birth. Preterm babies are at particular risk of hypothermia, and they should be delivered in a warm room and enclosed in clean plastic wrap before resuscitation to help maintain normothermia.

Intrauterine growth retardation

A baby with a birth weight below the 10th centile is small for gestational age (SGA). This may be familial or may be due to intrauterine growth retardation (IUGR). The pattern of growth retardation gives some indication of the cause. An insult in early pregnancy, such as infection, will cause symmetrical growth retardation. A later insult, usually placental insufficiency, will cause asymmetric growth retardation with relative sparing of head growth due to selective shunting of blood to the developing brain. Abnormalities of blood flow in the umbilical or fetal vessels can now be detected using Doppler ultrasound; these can be used to plan when to intervene and deliver the baby.

Causes of IUGR include:
• Multiple pregnancy
• Placental insufficiency
• Maternal smoking
• Congenital infections (e.g. toxoplasmosis, rubella)
• Genetic syndromes (e.g. Down's syndrome).

Babies with severe IUGR should be screened for congenital infection—'TORCH' screen (Toxoplasmosis, Other [syphilis], Rubella, Cytomegalovirus, Hepatitis, HIV). In the first few days of life, babies with IUGR are at risk of hypoglycaemia and hypothermia due to low glycogen stores and lack of subcutaneous fat. Symptomatic hypoglycaemia can cause neurodevelopmental injury. If there has been poor head growth during pregnancy, intellect may be impaired. Babies with IUGR must not be over-fed during infancy as there is evidence that excessive weight gain leads to hypertension, ischaemic heart disease and diabetes in later life.

Vitamin K

Vitamin K deficiency or persistent obstructive jaundice can lead to poor synthesis of vitamin K-dependent clotting factors and subsequent bleeding. The bleeding may be minor bruising or significant intracranial haemorrhage. This used to be known as haemorrhagic disease of the newborn but is now referred to as vitamin K deficiency bleeding (VKDB). Breast milk is low in vitamin K, unlike formula milk which is supplemented. For this reason vitamin K should be given routinely to all newborn infants, either as a single intramuscular injection or by mouth at birth, 1 and 6 weeks. Babies with persistent jaundice should receive further doses (see Chapter 48).

KEY POINTS

• Most babies are born healthy and do not require any resuscitation.
• The Apgar score is used to describe the condition after birth.
• Vitamin K is recommended for all babies.
• Babies with severe IUGR are at increased risk of asphyxia, hypoglycaemia and hypothermia, and may be at risk of intellectual impairment.

The newborn examination

All newborn babies are carefully examined in the first 24 h of life to check that they are healthy and to detect congenital abnormalities, some of which may not be obvious to the parents. The baby should be fully undressed in a warm room and examined from head to toe. Ask the mother if she has any concerns and whether there is any family history of note, for example of deafness or congenital dislocation of the hips

General observation
- Weight, length and head circumference
- Maturity
- Muscle tone
- Reflexes: Moro, grasp, suck and rooting
- Is this a healthy baby who is feeding well?

Face—dysmorphic features?
- Low set or simple ears
- Inner epicanthic folds
- Mongolian or anti-Mongolian slant of eyes
- Symmetry of face and mouth
- Accessory auricles and pre-auricular pits
- Micrognathia (small chin)

Heart
- Cyanosis
- Heart failure (tachypnoea, hepatomegaly)
- Heart murmur
- Femoral pulses (coarctation)
- Apex beat (dextrocardia)

Back and spine
- Spina bifida or posterior encephalocele
- Midline naevus, lipoma or deep sacral pit can suggest an underlying spinal abnormality

Hips
- Barlow and Ortolani tests for congenital dislocation of the hips (CDH)
- Ask about risk factors (breech, family history of CDH)

Genitalia and anus
- Hypospadias (urinary meatus on underside of penis)
- Cryptorchidism (undescended testes)
- Ambiguous genitalia: if both testes are impalpable, consider whether the baby could be a virilized female, due to congenital adrenal hypoplasia
- Imperforate anus (may have fistula to bladder or vagina)

Skin
- Pallor
- Jaundice
- Cyanosis
- Rashes (erythema toxicum is normal)
- Birthmarks (see Chapter 51)

Limbs
- Talipes equinovarus (club foot)
- Polydactyly (extra digits or toes)
- Syndactyly (fused digits or toes)
- Single palmar crease and 'sandal gap' between toes (Down's syndrome)
- Contractures (oligohydramnios or congenital muscular disorder)
- Absent radii (VACTERL association)

Head
- Anterior fontanelle
- Cephalhaematoma (parietal swelling that does not cross suture lines)
- Chignon from ventouse suction cup

Eyes
- Red reflex (to exclude cataract)
- Sclera (for jaundice)
- Coloboma (defect in the pupil)

Mouth
- Cleft lip/palate
- Central cyanosis
- Neonatal teeth

Chest
- Respiratory rate
- Respiratory distress
- Symmetry of chest movement (pneumothorax, diaphragmatic hernia)

Abdomen
- Abdominal distension or bile-stained vomiting suggest bowel obstruction
- Palpable kidneys (hydronephrosis)
- Anterior abdominal wall defects (gastroschisis or exomphalos)
- Three vessels in umbilical cord? (normal)

Common syndromes to be aware of:
- Trisomy 21 (Down's syndrome)
- Trisomy 13 (Patau's syndrome)
- Trisomy 18 (Edwards' syndrome)
- Turner's syndrome (45 XO)
- Noonan's syndrome (lymphoedema)
- VATER and VACTERL association
- Pierre Robin sequence

Patterns of congenital abnormality

The incidence of congenital abnormalities is 10–15 per 1000 births. The commonest are congenital heart defects (8 per 1000) (see Chapter 19). Abnormalities range from a trivial birth mark to a syndrome diagnosis. The majority of congenital abnormalities are genetically determined, but some may be due a combination of genetics and environment (e.g. spina bifida) or due entirely to environment (e.g. fetal alcohol syndrome).

A *syndrome* is a consistent pattern of dysmorphic features seen together, and suggests a genetic origin. A *sequence* is where one abnormality leads to another—for example, the small mandible (micrognathia) in Pierre Robin sequence causes posterior displacement of the tongue, which prevents the palate forming correctly, leading to cleft palate. An *association* is a non-random collection of abnormalities (see below).

Syndromes and associations

Syndromes	
Down's syndrome	Trisomy 21: See Chapters 8 and 63
Patau's syndrome	Trisomy 13 Midline defects, cleft lip and palate, cutis aplasia, holoprosencephaly, polydactyly, heart defects (VSD, PDA, ASD)
Edward's syndrome	Trisomy 18 IUGR, polyhydramnios, rocker-bottom feet, clenched hands, prominent occiput, heart defects (VSD, PDA, ASD), apnoea
Turner's syndrome	(45XO) See chapter 8.
Noonan's syndrome	Phenotypically similar to Turner's but occurs in both sexes. Short stature, oedema, pulmonary stenosis
Associations	
VACTERL	Vertebral, anal atresia, cardiac, tracheo-oesophageal fistula, renal, limb (absent radii)
CHARGE	Coloboma, heart defects, choanal atresia, retarded growth and development, genital hypoplasia and ear anomalies

Cleft lip and palate

Cleft lip occurs in 1 in 1000 infants. 70% have a cleft lip as well. Cleft lip may be diagnosed antenatally, allowing the parents to receive counselling. After birth a cleft palate is confirmed by palpating and observing the defect in the palate. A submucosal cleft is palpable but not visible. Cleft palate is best managed by a multidisciplinary team including plastic surgeon, orthodontist and speech therapist. Repair of the lip is performed at 3 months and the palate at 9 months. The cosmetic appearance following plastic surgery is excellent. Showing the parents 'before and after' photographs (see figure) can help allay anxiety. Expected difficulties include feeding difficulty, milk aspiration, conductive hearing loss and speech and dental problems. Regular audiological assessments are essential.

Neural tube defects ▸ (spina bifida)

Failure of the neural tube to close normally in early pregnancy causes spina bifida. It used to be a major cause of disability, but folic acid supplementation in early pregnancy has reduced the incidence by 75%. Antenatal ultrasound screening and selective termination has made open spina bifida a rare condition. Neural tube defects are always midline. The severity depends on the extent to which the neural tube has failed to develop:
• **Anencephaly.** The cranial part of the neural tube does not exist and the brain cortex does not develop. Infants die soon after birth.

a) Cleft lip (before surgery)   **b) Cleft lip repaired**

Source: Queen Victoria Hospital NHS Foundation Trust

• **Myelomeningocele.** An open lesion where the spinal cord is covered by a thin membrane of meninges. There is severe weakness of the lower limbs with bladder and anal denervation and an associated hydrocephalus. Survivors have severe disability.
• **Meningocele.** The spinal cord is intact but there is an exposed sac of meninges which can rupture, with the risk of meningitis.
• **Spina bifida occulta.** A 'hidden' neural tube defect where the vertebral bodies fail to fuse posteriorly. Some degree may be present in 5–10% of normal infants. The only clue may be a tuft of hair, naevus, lipoma or deep sacral pit in the midline over the lower back. A spinal ultrasound is indicated.

▸ Developmental dysplasia of the hip

Developmental dysplasia of the hip (DDH) occurs in 1% of infants. The acetabulum is shallow and does not adequately cover the femoral head, leading to the hip joint being, dislocatable or dislocated. Risk factors are breech position, family history, female sex and impaired limb movement. There is an association with talipes. True congenital dislocation of the hip (CDH) occurs in 2 per 1000 infants. Examination includes observation of symmetrical skin creases and leg length, the Ortolani test (a *dislocated* hip will not abduct fully, and 'clunks' as it relocates into the acetabulum) and the Barlow test (feeling a clunk as a *dislocatable* hip slips out of the acetabulum). Babies with risk factors or abnormal examination should have an ultrasound of the hip joint before 12 weeks. Treatment involves wearing a harness or splint to hold the joint in flexion and abduction for several months.

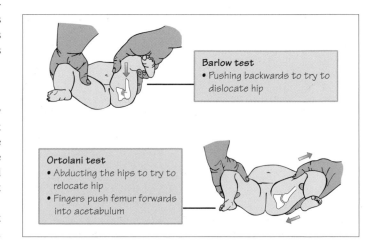

Barlow test
• Pushing backwards to try to dislocate hip

Ortolani test
• Abducting the hips to try to relocate hip
• Fingers push femur forwards into acetabulum

Screening and genetics

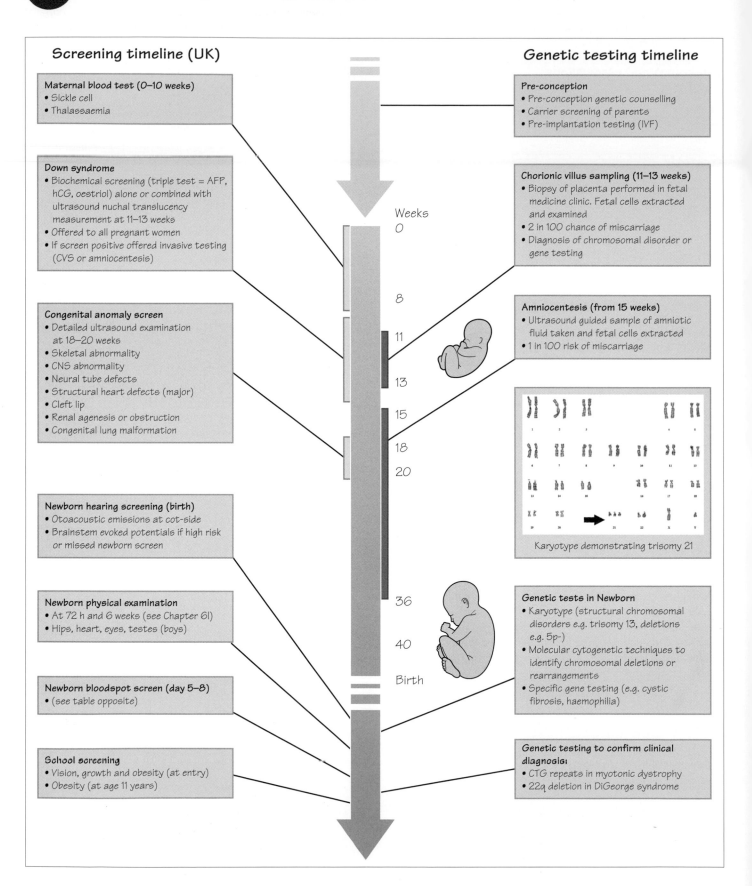

Screening timeline (UK)

Maternal blood test (0–10 weeks)
• Sickle cell
• Thalassaemia

Down syndrome
• Biochemical screening (triple test = AFP, hCG, oestriol) alone or combined with ultrasound nuchal translucency measurement at 11–13 weeks
• Offered to all pregnant women
• If screen positive offered invasive testing (CVS or amniocentesis)

Congenital anomaly screen
• Detailed ultrasound examination at 18–20 weeks
• Skeletal abnormality
• CNS abnormality
• Neural tube defects
• Structural heart defects (major)
• Cleft lip
• Renal agenesis or obstruction
• Congenital lung malformation

Newborn hearing screening (birth)
• Otoacoustic emissions at cot-side
• Brainstem evoked potentials if high risk or missed newborn screen

Newborn physical examination
• At 72 h and 6 weeks (see Chapter 61)
• Hips, heart, eyes, testes (boys)

Newborn bloodspot screen (day 5–8)
• (see table opposite)

School screening
• Vision, growth and obesity (at entry)
• Obesity (at age 11 years)

Genetic testing timeline

Pre-conception
• Pre-conception genetic counselling
• Carrier screening of parents
• Pre-implantation testing (IVF)

Chorionic villus sampling (11–13 weeks)
• Biopsy of placenta performed in fetal medicine clinic. Fetal cells extracted and examined
• 2 in 100 chance of miscarriage
• Diagnosis of chromosomal disorder or gene testing

Amniocentesis (from 15 weeks)
• Ultrasound guided sample of amniotic fluid taken and fetal cells extracted
• 1 in 100 risk of miscarriage

Karyotype demonstrating trisomy 21

Genetic tests in Newborn
• Karyotype (structural chromosomal disorders e.g. trisomy 13, deletions e.g. 5p-)
• Molecular cytogenetic techniques to identify chromosomal deletions or rearrangements
• Specific gene testing (e.g. cystic fibrosis, haemophilia)

Genetic testing to confirm clinical diagnosis:
• CTG repeats in myotonic dystrophy
• 22q deletion in DiGeorge syndrome

Weeks
0
8
11
13
15
18
20
36
40
Birth

 Paediatrics at a Glance, Third Edition. Lawrence Miall, Mary Rudolf, Dominic Smith. © 2012 John Wiley & Sons, Ltd. Published 2012 by John Wiley & Sons, Ltd.

Screening

Screening aims to identify unrecognized disease in apparently well people. Cost must be considered and balanced against that of treatment if the problem presents later. Conditions suitable for screening should:
- Be identifiable at a latent or early symptomatic stage
- Be treatable.
- Have a better prognosis if treated early.

Screening of newborns and children in the UK is outlined opposite and in the box below. Further information is available at http://www.screening.nhs.uk/england.

Genetic disorders

Most disorders that are screened for in newborns have a genetic basis. Molecular genetic techniques are increasingly used to identify abnormal genes or chromosomes. It is vital that families receive appropriate counselling so that they understand the implications of an abnormal result. Genetic tests can be performed at various times:
- **Pre-implantation testing** is only available with in-vitro fertilization techniques, but can allow screening prior to implantation.
- **Antenatal genetic testing** via chorionic villus sampling or amniocentesis allows the possibility of termination of pregnancy. Some families choose to continue the pregnancy despite a positive result and this allows them time to come to terms with the diagnosis.
- **Newborn genetic testing** may be performed to confirm a clinical diagnosis (e.g. Down's syndrome or congenital myotonic dystrophy) or following a positive screening test (e.g. CF gene testing following an abnormal IRT result on the newborn blood spot screen).
- **Genetic testing of older children** may be needed to confirm a diagnosis presenting later in childhood (e.g. fragile X or Duchenne muscular dystrophy). In general children must not be tested for adult-onset genetic disorders without their own informed consent unless it is going to alter their treatment during childhood.

Genetic inheritance

Many genetic disorders occur sporadically with no preceding family history or are multifactorial, with an environmental element (e.g. diabetes), but some single-gene disorders show a clear inheritance pattern:
- **Autosomal recessive:** both parents carry an abnormal copy of the gene (carrier). 25% of their children will inherit both abnormal genes and be affected. 50% of offspring inherit one abnormal gene and are themselves carriers and usually unaffected. 25% of offspring do not inherit either abnormal gene.
- **Autosomal dominant:** inheriting even a single copy of the abnormal gene from either parent means the child is affected. These conditions sometimes present earlier or more severely in successive generations (anticipation). Sometimes the effect of a gene mutation will depend on which parent it is inherited from (imprinting).
- **Sex-linked inheritance:** gene disorders on the X chromosome usually only present in boys, as the presence of a second normal X chromosome in girls prevent them being severely affected. Examples include haemophilia A and fragile X syndrome.
- **Chromosomal disorders:** these are usually sporadic due to non-disjunction of chromosomes during meiosis (trisomy 21, 18 or 13) or due to rearrangement of major parts of the chromosome (translocations). In Turner's syndrome there is deletion of one X chromosome (45 XO). In some cases there is deletion of part of a chromosome, e.g. cri du chat syndrome (5p- deletion).

Screening for Down's syndrome

Down's syndrome affects 1 in 1000 live births (1 in 600 fetuses). There is an association with increased maternal age (1 in 880 at 30 years rising to 1 in 100 at age 40 years). 95% are due to non-disjunction during meiosis and 3% to an unbalanced translocation. 1% are mosaics, with only a proportion of cells within the body having trisomy 21. About 55% of affected fetuses are detected antenatally, through screening. In those diagnosed antenatally, only 5% of couples choose to continue with the pregnancy. Antenatal screening involves measurement of AFP, hCG and oestriol (the 'triple' test) and other markers, with nuchal fold (subcutaneous tissue at back of the neck) thickness in the fetus. This gives a calculated risk, which if high may prompt diagnostic testing via chorionic villus sampling or amniocentesis.

Notes
The midwife will collect bloodspots from the heel of every newborn baby on day 5–8 of life on to an absorbent card. These are analysed and also stored for further diagnostic tests if necessary

Congenital hypothyroidism	Screen detects high TSH level but will miss hypothyroidism secondary to pituitary dysfunction. Thyroid replacement allows normal development
▶ Sickle cell disease	Universal screening to all pregnant women aims to identify at-risk couples. Newborn bloodspots are analysed by HPLC for all sickle cell variants
Phenyketonuria (PKU)	A phenylalanine assay has replaced the original 'Guthrie' test. Babies PKU need urgent advice on starting a low-phenylalanine diet and long-term follow-up to prevent learning disability from phenylalanine metabolites
▶ Cystic fibrosis (CF)	A high immunoreactive trypsin (IRT) on the newborn blood spot is followed up with DNA testing for common CF mutations
Medium-chain acylcarnitine deficiency (MCAD)	A fatty acid oxidation defect that can lead to significant hypoglycaemia during periods of illness. Acylcarnitine abnormalities can be detected by tandem mass spectrometry. MCAD is a preventable cause of sudden death in infancy. Frequent feeds prevent the need for breakdown of fatty acids

Complications of prematurity

Eyes
- Retinopathy of prematurity due to abnormal vascularization of the developing retina
- Require laser treatment to prevent retinal detachment and blindness

Respiratory
- Respiratory distress syndrome (surfactant deficiency)
- Apnoea and bradycardia
- Pneumothorax
- Chronic lung disease

Cardiovascular (see Chapter 19)
- Hypotension
- Patent ductus arteriosus

Temperature control
- Increased surface area to volume ratio leads to loss of heat
- Immature skin cannot retain heat and fluid efficiently
- Reduced subcutaneous fat reduces insulation

Metabolic
- Hypoglycaemia is common. Symptomatic hypoglycaemia must be treated promptly. Blood glucose should be maintained above 2.6 mmol/L to prevent neurological damage
- Hypocalcaemia
- Electrolyte imbalance
- Osteopenia of prematurity (with risk of fractures)

Brain
- Intraventricular haemorrhage
- Posthaemorrhagic hydrocephalus
- Periventricular leucomalacia
- Increased risk of cerebral palsy

Nutrition
- May require parenteral nutrition
- Nasogastric feeds until sucking reflex develops at 32–34 weeks
- Difficult to achieve in-utero growth rates

Gastrointestinal
- Necrotizing enterocolitis: a life-threatening inflammation of the bowel wall due to ischaemia and infection and which can lead to bowel perforation
- Gastro-oesophageal reflux
- Inguinal hernias (with high risk of strangulation)

Infection
- Increased risk of sepsis, especially group B streptococcus and coliforms
- Pneumonia is common
- Infection is a common complication of central venous lines required for feeding

Blood
- Anaemia of prematurity
- Neonatal jaundice (see Chapter 48)

What you need from your evaluation

History

- **Risk factors for prematurity:** young maternal age, multiple pregnancy, infection, maternal illness (e.g. pregnancy-induced hypertension), cervical incompetence, antepartum haemorrhage, smoking, alcohol and infection
- **Full obstetric history**
- **Condition at birth:** Apgar score, resuscitation required
- **Birthweight:** appropriate for gestational age?
- **Gestation:** must be known to give accurate prognosis. Calculate from menstrual period, by early dating ultrasound scan or by assessment of gestation after birth (Dubowitz score)
  Associated problems such as twin pregnancy (much higher risk of poor neurological outcome), congenital abnormalities or infection (chorioamnionitis may have been trigger for preterm labour)
- **Antenatal steroids:** if given, these reduce the incidence of respiratory distress syndrome and intraventricular haemorrhage

Long-term complications

- **Survival:** about 45% of infants born alive at 24 weeks gestation survive. By 27 weeks this rises to 80% and after 32 weeks the chances of survival are excellent
- **Chronic lung disease** (bronchopulmonary dysplasia): this is a consequence of disrupted lung development and may require long-term oxygen treatment for months or sometimes years
- **Neurological sequelae:** there is a significant risk of hydrocephalus developing secondary to an intraventricular haemorrhage. A shunt may need to be inserted to relieve pressure. Hypotension may have been sustained, leading to periventricular leucomalacia. This carries the risk of cerebral palsy, particularly of the diplegic type
- **Blindness:** as a consequence of severe retinopathy of prematurity (ROP). This is becoming less common with better prevention, detection and treatment of ROP
- **Poor growth:** especially if catch-up growth is not achieved

7% of all babies are premature (<37 weeks) and 1% are extremely premature (<28 weeks) or very low birthweight (VLBW<1500 g). Premature babies can survive from 23–24 weeks gestation, although mortality is high (25% survival at 23 weeks, 45% at 24 weeks) and only 25% of those that survive at these gestations will be free of disability. Beyond 30–32 weeks the prognosis is excellent. Premature infants are at risk of complications such as hypothermia, hypoglycaemia and difficulty feeding, which are common to IUGR babies too.

Premature babies need care on a special care baby unit (SCBU) or neonatal intensive care unit (NICU). Incubators provide warmth and humidity to prevent hypothermia and protect the skin, which is thin, red and transparent and does not provide an adequate barrier to heat and fluid loss. Feeding problems are common. A mature suck–swallow pattern does not develop until 34 weeks, so premature babies need to be fed via a nasogastric tube. Very sick premature babies, or those with IUGR or asphyxia, may be at increased risk of necrotizing enterocolitis (NEC) and are therefore given intravenous parenteral nutrition. Premature babies are at risk of infection, either acquired from the mother during delivery or from the hospital environment and to brain injury (see below).

▶ Respiratory distress syndrome

Pneumonia, pneumothorax, cardiac failure and congenital lung malformation can all cause respiratory distress in preterm infants but by far the commonest cause is respiratory distress syndrome (RDS) due to surfactant deficiency.

Signs of RDS include tachypnoea, intercostal recession, cyanosis and expiratory 'grunting'. CXR shows a 'ground glass' appearance due to alveolar collapse with an air-bronchogram. RDS is caused by lack of surfactant, a phospholipid which reduces alveolar surface tension. Surfactant production is not mature until about 35–36 weeks, although the stress of labour usually stimulates production, and RDS is therefore usually self-limiting, lasting 5–7 days. Corticosteroids administered antenatally to at risk mothers reduce RDS by stimulating surfactant production. IUGR babies are physiologically 'stressed' and tend to get less severe RDS due to endogenous corticosteroid release.

Management involves optimizing oxygenation and supporting respiration, either with continuous positive airway pressure (CPAP) via nasal prongs, or by mechanical ventilation. Surfactant can be administered via an endotracheal tube. This treatment has reduced the mortality of RDS by over 40%. 20% of babies with RDS develop chronic lung disease of prematurity (bronchopulmonary dysplasia) which if severe may require home-oxygen therapy.

▶ Necrotizing enterocolitis

This serious complication is due to impaired blood flow to the bowel. Mucosal ischaemia allows gut microorganisms to penetrate the bowel wall causing a severe haemorrhagic colitis. Breast milk is protective, but increasing milk feeds (especially formula feeds) too rapidly is a risk factor for NEC, as is a patent arterial duct (PDA). NEC presents with acute collapse, abdominal distension, bile-stained vomiting and bloody diarrhoea. An abdominal radiograph may show gas in the bowel wall or portal veins. Management involves stopping feeds, supporting the circulation and antibiotics. Laparotomy is required if perforation occurs. Complications include intestinal stricture and short bowel syndrome.

Retinopathy of prematurity

Retinopathy of prematurity (ROP) is common in very premature infants, occurring in up to 35% of VLBW babies. In most cases it

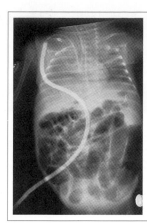

Dilated bowel loops and intramural gas typical of NEC. There is a central venous line and a nasogastric tube in place

requires no treatment but in about 1% of these babies it causes blindness. ROP is caused by proliferation of new blood vessels in an area of relative ischaemia in the developing retina. Oxygen toxicity is one cause although there may also be a genetic predisposition. At-risk infants should be screened for ROP by an ophthalmologist. If detected, laser ablation can be used to prevent the risk of retinal detachment and blindness.

▶ Brain injury

Preterm infants are at risk of brain injury and this is the most important factor affecting their long-term prognosis. Periventricular leucomalacia, large intraventricular haemorrhage and post-haemorrhagic hydrocephalus are the most important lesions causing disability.

• **Intraventricular haemorrhage** (IVH) occurs in up to 30% of VLBW. Haemorrhage develops in the floor of the lateral ventricle and ruptures into the ventricle. In a small minority the haemorrhage involves the white matter around the ventricle by a process of obstructive venous infarction. This carries a high risk of hemiplegic cerebral palsy (see Chapter 42). IVH may be asymptomatic and is diagnosed by cerebral ultrasound scan.

• **Posthaemorrhagic hydrocephalus** occurs in 15% of severe IVH and may require insertion of a ventriculo-peritoneal shunt.

• **Periventricular leucomalacia** is caused by ischaemic damage to the periventricular white matter. It is less common than IVH, but is the commonest cause of cerebral palsy in surviving infants. PVL is particularly likely where there has been chorioamnionitis, severe hypotension or in monozygotic twins. The prognosis is worse if cystic change develops, with 80% developing cerebral palsy.

Neurodevelopment

There is an increased incidence of learning difficulties in extremely preterm infants. Attention difficulties are common, and subtle problems in higher functioning may not manifest until school age.

KEY POINTS

• 7% of infants are born before <37 weeks. 1% are extremely premature <28 weeks.
• Complications relate to organ immaturity and include hypothermia, hypoglycaemia and surfactant deficient RDS.
• Premature babies are at increased risk of cerebral palsy due to intracranial haemorrhage and white matter injury.
• Perinatal infection (chorioamnionitis) is an important risk factor for preterm labour and for cerebral palsy.

Breast-feeding

Ways to encourage successful breast-feeding
- Introduce concept of breast-feeding to both parents antenatally
- Put the baby to the breast immediately after delivery
- Allow the baby to feed on demand, especially in the early days
- Avoid offering any formula feeds
- Ensure mother receives good nutrition and plenty of rest
- Provide skilled breast-feeding advisors to help mother through any initial problems with breast-feeding
- Ensure correct 'latching on' with the baby's mouth wide open and good positioning

Lactation
- At birth, prolactin levels rise sharply and this is further stimulated by the infant sucking at the breast. Prolactin determines milk production from the breast alveoli, and is increased by the frequency, duration and intensity of sucking
- The actual flow of milk is aided by the 'let-down' reflex. Rooting at the nipple causes afferent pathways to stimulate the posterior pituitary to secrete oxytocin, which stimulates the smooth muscle around the alveolar ducts to express the milk from the breast. The let-down reflex can be stimulated by hearing the baby cry or by contact with the baby, and can be inhibited by stress or embarrassment
- The majority of the milk is taken from the breast in the first 5 min and this may be followed by non-nutritive sucking

Advantages of breast-feeding
- Perfect balance of milk constituents
- Little risk of bacterial contamination
- Anti-infective properties (IgA, macrophages, etc.)
- Ideal food for brain growth and development
- Convenient
- No expense of purchasing milk
- Psychologically satisfying
- Reduces risk of atopic disorders

Possible problems with breast-feeding (rare)
- Can initially be tiring for the mother
- Can transmit infection (e.g. HIV, although in developing countries the best advice is still to exclusively breast-feed)
- Some drugs can be excreted in breast milk (e.g. warfarin)

Weaning
- 0–6 months: breast or formula milk only
- 6 months: puréed or liquidized foods
- 7–9 months: finger foods, juice in a cup
- 9–12 months: 3 meals a day with family and 3 snacktimes
- >1 year: cow's milk in a beaker or cup; adult-type food chopped up

Formula milk feeds

- Formula milks are based on cow's milk, but are carefully adjusted to meet the basic nutritional requirements of growing infants. The fat component is generally replaced with polyunsaturated vegetable oils to provide the correct essential fatty acids. Minerals, vitamins and trace elements are then added
- Formula milk is usually made up from a dry powder, by adding one level measure of powder to each 30 mL (1 fl.oz) of cooled boiled water. Great care must be taken to sterilize the bottles and teats carefully to avoid introducing infection. The milk is then re-warmed prior to feeding. Ensure the milk is at a safe comfortable temperature before feeding. Never re-warm in a microwave. Each feed should be made freshly.

1. Sterilize the feeding bottle
2. Add the appropriate volume of cooled boiled water to the bottle
3. Add 1 level scoop of milk powder to each 30 mL of water
4. Shake bottle well
5. Ensure the milk is at a safe comfortable temperature before feeding

Infant nutrition

Milk provides all the nutrients needed by newborn infants for the first 6 months of life. Breast milk is the ideal milk for human babies, but formula milk may be needed as an alternative in some cases. The newborn infant has high calorie and fluid requirements and to achieve optimal growth requires approximately 150 mL/kg per day of fluid and 110 kcal/kg per day (462 kJ/kg per day). About 40% of this energy comes from carbohydrate (mostly lactose) and 50% from fat. Milk also contains protein in the form of casein, lactalbumin and lactoferrin. Colostrum is the thin yellow milk produced in the first few days which is high in immunoglobulins.

Infants also require adequate amounts of minerals such as calcium and phosphate, as well as vitamins and trace elements. Breast milk is deficient in vitamin K, and so all newborn infants are given vitamin K at birth to prevent haemorrhagic disease of the newborn. Weaning on to solids usually starts around 6 months, and infants should not have cow's milk until they are over a year.

The stool pattern of breast-fed babies differs from that of bottle-fed babies. They have non-offensive, porridge-consistency, yellow stools, initially after each feed. The frequency then reduces so they may have only one per week without being constipated.

Technique of breast-feeding

Mothers should be encouraged to put their babies to the breast soon after delivery. Little milk is produced but the suckling stimulates lactation. Colostrum is produced in the first days, which is rich in energy and anti-infective agents. It is important that the baby is taught to 'latch on' to the breast properly with a widely open mouth, so that the areola and not just the nipple is within the baby's mouth. The majority of the milk is taken by the baby in the first 5 minutes. Time after this is spent in non-nutritive suckling. Mothers can feel their breast 'emptying'. Babies should not be pulled off the breast, but the suck released by inserting a clean finger at the side of the baby's mouth. Each feed should start on the alternate breast.

In the first few days the breasts may become painfully engorged with milk and the nipples sore, especially if the baby's position is not optimal. Mothers need a lot of encouragement and advice to get through this time.

It is important to try to avoid alternating breast and formula feeds. Formula feeds should only be introduced if breast-feeding is contraindicated or has failed completely. It is not appropriate to 'top up' with formula or use bottles to give the mother a rest. This may help in the short term but leads to tailing off of milk production and breast-feeding failing altogether.

Weaning

Current recommendations are to start weaning at 6 months of age. Generally cereals, rusks or rice-based mixtures are introduced first, mixed with expressed breast milk or formula milk. This semi-solid mixture can be given by spoon before milk feeds. Puréed fruit or vegetables are also suitable. Modern baby cereals are gluten-free, which may be associated with a fall in the incidence of coeliac disease (see p. 000). As the child grows older the feeds can become more solid and are given as three meals a day. From 7 to 9 months they will enjoy finger-feeding themselves and can chew on rusks or toast. From about 9 months they can generally eat a mashed or cut-up version of adult food. Undiluted full-fat pasteurized cow's milk can be given from 1 year of age. An earlier introduction of cow's milk or the persistence of exclusive breast-feeding can lead to iron deficiency. Vitamin supplements may be needed from 6 months in breast-fed babies, until they are on a full mixed diet.

Nutrition in the preschool years

As a toddler the child becomes more adept at holding a spoon and can feed independently, and can drink from a beaker or cup. Milk is no longer the main source of nutrients, although the child should still drink a pint a day. Whole-fat milk should be used until age 5 years to provide plenty of calories, unless the child is overweight. A well-balanced diet should include food from the four main groups:

- Meat, fish, poultry and eggs
- Dairy products (milk, cheese, yoghurt)
- Fruit and vegetables
- Cereals, grains, potatoes and rice.

In order to avoid dental caries and obesity it is important to avoid frequent snacking on sugary foods or drinks—three meals and two snacks is recommended, although this may be adapted to the individual child. Iron-deficiency anaemia (see Chapter 47) is common at this age, due to high requirements for growth and poor dietary intake, especially in the 'faddy eater'. Vitamin C present in orange juice can enhance iron absorption from the gut.

Nutrition in the school-age child

At school, children have to learn to eat food outside the family setting. They usually have a midday meal, and fruit or milk may be provided at break times. The principles of healthy eating should be maintained, although peer pressure to eat crisps or sugary snacks is often high. Schools have an educational role to play in encouraging healthy eating and a healthy lifestyle. During adolescence there is a greater energy requirement to allow for increased growth. This may coincide with a lifestyle that leads to snacking and missing meals, or to restrictive dieting or the over-consumption of fast food. Obesity and eating disorders often have their onset around this time.

KEY POINTS

- Breast milk provides ideal nutrition for babies.
- The optimum time for weaning is 6 months.
- Formula feeds need to be made up carefully to avoid infection.
- 'Doorstep' cow's milk should not be used until 1 year.
- Full-fat milk is recommended until 5 years of age.
- Toddlers need to be allowed to explore food and develop independent eating habits.

Common behaviour problems

The crying baby
- Wet or dirty nappy
- Too hot or too cold
- Hungry
- Wind
- Colic
- Environmental stress
- Reflux oesophagitis
- Teething

If sudden severe crying, consider:
- Any acute illness
- Otitis media
- ►Intussusception
- ►Strangulated inguinal hernia

Temper tantrums
- Normal, peak at 18–36 months
- Screaming
- Hitting
- Biting
- Breath-holding attacks (see Chapter 40)

Strategies that may help
- Avoid precipitants such as hunger and tiredness
- Divert the tantrum by distraction
- Stay calm to teach control
- Reward good behaviour
- Try to ignore bad behaviour until calm
- Use time-out

Sleeping problems
- Difficulty getting to sleep
- Waking during the night
- Sleeping in parents' bed
- Nightmares and night terrors

Eating problems in toddlers
- Food refusal
- Fussy eating—only eating a limited variety of foods
- Overeating
- Battles over eating and mealtimes
- Snacking
- Excessive drinking of juice

Unwanted habits
- Thumb sucking
- Nail biting
- Masturbation
- Head banging
- Hair pulling
- Bedwetting
- Encopresis (passing faeces in inappropriate places)

Aggressive behaviour
- Temper tantrums
- Hitting and biting other children
- Destroying toys
- Destroying furniture
- Commoner in boys and in larger families
- May reflect aggression within family
- Requires calm, consistent approach
- Avoid countering with aggression
- Use time-out and star charts

What you need from your evaluation

History
- Ask what is troubling the parents most—is it the child or other stresses in their lives, such as tiredness, problems at work or relationship problems?
- What are the triggers for difficult or unwanted behaviour? Does it occur when the child is hungry or tired, or at any particular time of day?
- Colic tends to occur in the evenings; tantrums may be more common if the child is tired
- Does the behaviour happen consistently in all settings or is it specific to one place, e.g. the toddler may behave well at nursery but show difficult behaviour at home?
- Does the behaviour differ with each parent?
- How do the parents deal with the behaviour—do they get angry or aggressive, are they consistent, do they use bribery or do they give in to the toddler eventually?
- What strategies have the parents already tried to deal with the situation?
- Is there any serious risk of harm? Some behaviour, such as encopresis or deliberate self-harm, may reflect serious emotional upset. Most toddlers who are faddy eaters are growing well and do not suffer any long-term nutritional problems
- Babies with colic are usually less than 3 months old, go red in the face with a tense abdomen and draw up their legs. The episodes start abruptly and end with the passage of flatus or faeces

Examination
- The history usually contributes more than a physical examination
- If the parents are concerned about sudden-onset or severe crying in a baby, it is important to exclude serious infection such as meningitis or urinary tract infection, intussusception, hernias and otitis media

Management
- In most cases the parents can be reassured that the behaviour is very common, often normal and that with time and common sense it can be controlled
- With tantrums it can be helpful to use the ABC approach:
  - A What **a**ntecedents were there? What happened to trigger the episode?
  - B What was the **b**ehaviour? Could it be modified, diverted or stopped?
  - C What were the **c**onsequences of the behaviour? Was the child told off, shouted at or given a cuddle?
- Generally, it is best to reward good behaviour (catch the child being good) and ignore bad behaviour. Star charts can be very useful: the child gets a star for good behaviour (staying in bed, etc.) and then a reward after several stars
- Parents should try hard not to be angry or aggressive as this may reinforce attention-seeking behaviour

Common emotional and behavioural problems

These problems are seen so often that many would regard them as normal, although in a small minority the behaviour is so disruptive that it causes major family upset. General practitioners and paediatricians should be comfortable giving basic guidance on behaviour management to help parents through what can be a stressful, exasperating and exhausting phase of their child's development.

Crying babies and colic

Crying is usually periodic and related to discomfort, stress or temperament. However, it may indicate a serious problem, particularly if the onset is sudden. In most instances it is just a case of ensuring that the baby is well fed, warm but not too hot, has a clean nappy, comfortable clothes and a calm and peaceful environment. A persistently crying baby can be very stressful for inexperienced parents. It is important that they recognize when they are no longer coping and are offered support.

▶ **Infantile colic** is a term used to describe periodic crying affecting infants in the first 3 months of life. The crying is paroxysmal, and may be associated with hunger, swallowed air or discomfort from overfeeding. It often occurs in the evenings. Crying can last for several hours, with a flushed face, distended and tense abdomen and drawn-up legs. In between attacks the child is happy and well. It is important to consider more serious pathology such as intussusception or infection. Colic is managed by giving advice on feeding, winding after feeds and carrying the baby. It is not a reason to stop breast-feeding, but discontinuing cow's milk in the mother's diet can be helpful. Various remedies are available but there is little evidence for their effectiveness. Infantile colic usually resolves spontaneously by 3 months.

▶ Feeding problems

Once weaned, infants need to gradually move from being fed with a spoon to finger feeding and feeding themselves. This is a messy time, but the infant needs to be allowed to explore their food and not be made to eat or reprimanded for making a mess.

Toddler eating habits can be unpredictable—eating large amounts at one meal and sometimes hardly anything at the next. At this age, mealtimes can easily become a battle and it is important that they are kept relaxed and the child is not pressurized into eating. Small helpings that the child can finish work best, and second helpings can be given if wanted. Eating together as a family encourages the child to eat in a social context. Feeding at mealtimes should not become a long protracted battle!

▶ Sleeping problems

Babies and children differ in the amount of sleep they need and parents vary in how they tolerate their child waking at night. In most cases sleeping 'difficulties' are really just habits that have developed through lack of clear bedtime routine. Difficulty sleeping may also reflect conflict in the family or anxieties, for example about starting school or fear of dying. Successfully tackling sleeping problems requires determination, support and reassurance.

• **Refusal to settle at night.** Difficulty settling may develop if babies are only put to bed once they are asleep. A clear bedtime routine is important for older children—for example a bath, a story and a drink.
• **Waking during the night.** This often causes a lot of stress as the parents become exhausted. It is important to reassure the child, then put them back to bed quietly. Sometimes a technique of 'controlled crying' can be helpful—the child is left to cry for a few minutes, then reassured and left again, this time for longer. Taking the child into the parents' bed is understandable, but usually stores up problems for later when it is difficult to break the habit.
• **Nightmares.** The child wakes as the result of a bad dream, quickly becomes lucid and can usually remember the content. The child should be reassured and returned to sleep. If particularly severe or persistent, nightmares may reflect stresses and may need psychological help.
• **Night terrors.** Night terrors occur in preschool years. The child wakes up confused, disorientated and frightened and may not recognize their parent. They take several minutes to become orientated and the dream content cannot be recalled. These episodes should not be confused with epilepsy. They are short-lived and just require reassurance, especially for the parents.

Temper tantrums

Tantrums are very common in the third year of life (the 'terrible twos') and are part of the child learning the boundaries of acceptable behaviour and parental control. They can be extremely challenging, especially when they occur in public!

The key to dealing with toddler tantrums is to try to avoid getting into the situation in the first place. This does not mean giving in to the child's every demand, but ensuring the child does not get overtired or hungry, and setting clear boundaries in a calm, consistent way. It is generally best to ignore the tantrum until the child calms down. If this fails then 'time out' can be a useful technique. The child is taken to a safe quiet environment, such as a bedroom, and left for a few minutes (1 minute for each year of age is a good guide) until calm. This is usually very effective as it removes the attention the child desires, and allows the parents time to control their own anger.

Unwanted or aggressive behaviour

Young children often have aggressive outbursts which may involve biting, hitting or scratching other children. These require consistent firm management, with use of time out and star charts for good behaviour. It is important not to respond with more aggression, as this sends conflicting messages. If aggressive behaviour is persistent it is important to explore other tensions or disturbances within the family. In older children, the school may need to be involved.

Unwanted behaviours such as thumb-sucking, hair-pulling, nail-biting and masturbation are also common in young children. The majority can be ignored and resolve with time. Masturbation can usually be prevented by distracting the child or dressing them in clothes that make it more difficult. Older children should not be reprimanded but informed that it is not acceptable in public.

KEY POINTS

• Emotional and behavioural problems are extremely common, to the point of being part of normal child development.
• Parents need to be encouraged that they can manage most behaviour with a clear strategy.
• A calm, confident consistent approach to the child's behaviour is recommended.
• Parents should reward good behaviour and try to minimize attention given to undesirable behaviour.

Child care

Increasingly, mothers are working outside the home and need to find care for their children. Options include:

- A nanny or minder
- A childminder who takes other children into their own home and has to be legally approved and registered with the social services
- A day nursery staffed by nursery nurses and run either privately, by social services departments, or by voluntary organizations
- Children's Centres are a new initiative in disadvantaged areas that provide a variety of facilities and programmes for young families

Education

Compulsory education begins at age 5 and continues to age 16. For younger children there are opportunities to meet, play and socialize with others

Preschool

- Mother and toddler groups for children accompanied by a carer
- Playgroups run by trained and registered leaders
- A limited availability of nursery school places from 3 years of age

School

- Primary school from 5 to 11 years of age
- Secondary school from 11 to 16 years
- Sixth form, sixth form college or college of further education at age 16 years

School and health

Health promotion

School offers the opportunity to educate children about healthy living

- healthy relationships
- nutrition
- physical activity
- drugs and alcohol abuse
- contraception and safe sex
- smoking
- parenting skills

The child with medical problems (see Chapter)

Doctors have a role in making sure that children who have chronic health problems are well integrated and that staff understand the child's medical condition

The child with special educational needs (see Chapter 63)

Where at all possible, children with special educational needs are included in mainstream education. One teacher (the SENCO) has responsibility for children with educational needs in the school. She ensures the child is supported through learning in small groups or with special needs assistance. When needed, physiotherapy, occupational therapy and speech and language therapy is provided at school

Common problems at school age
Attention deficit and hyperactivity disorder
Hyperactivity is characterised by overactivity, difficulty keeping still and restlessness. It can be so extreme as to impair learning and disrupt classes. These children can be impulsive and excitable. Children with *attention deficit disorder* have difficulty concentrating on a task. It may or may not occur with hyperactivity (when it is known as ADHD) and is more common in boys.

Diagnosis of ADHD requires independent reporting by family and school as well as direct observation of the child. The problems need to be pervasive (present in different settings). Management includes strategies to reduce distraction, focus on task, build concentration, and provision of a calm regular daily routine with consistent boundaries. Support with teaching assistance may be helpful to help the child focus on tasks. Central nervous system (CNS) stimulant drugs such as methylphenidate can help improve concentration but behavioural strategies are preferable.

Aggressive behaviour
Temper tantrums with shouting and physical outbursts are normal in the toddler years but should settle as children learn to control their anger and frustration through consistent parenting. Aggressive behaviour in children is very rarely caused by medical illness (e.g. precocious puberty, frontal lobe problems). It is most often behaviour that the child has learned from their home environment by adults showing verbal or physical aggression, for example if the child witnesses domestic violence. Aggressive children may be involved in bullying in school and further social problems beyond. If persistent then the description 'conduct disorder' is sometimes applied. Maintaining a calm environment with emotional warmth and clear boundaries at home is necessary. School staff should be involved along with parents in order to address peer problems, academic or social problems and to institute behaviour modification.

► Teasing and bullying
Bullying is when a child deliberately behaves in a way that upsets or frightens another child. This can be a single episode or repeated over long periods of time and can lead to significant distress. The bullied child may react by becoming withdrawn or aggressive, or may develop illness symptoms. In schools where bullying is a problem, a whole-school approach where both the victims and the bullies are helped is most effective. The bullied child needs to feel safe and supported if they disclose. They need help in handling the situation and to increase social confidence.

Non-attendance at school
Most absences from school occur as a result of acute illness, which is usually minor, but may be prolonged through parental anxiety. School refusal may be due to separation anxiety (common on first starting school) or school phobia (usually triggered by distressing events, such as problems with peers). There may be abnormal attachment affecting the parent–child relationship. The child may have non-specific illness symptoms and social withdrawal.

Truancy is most common at secondary school age. Persistent truancy is associated with antisocial behaviour, poor academic achievement and family relationship problems.

Management of both must involve close collaboration between the parents and teachers. The child should be supported in a gradual return to full school attendance through a combined approach between parents, school, child health and child psychology. Truancy is managed with school or education welfare staff.

Severe educational difficulties
Reasons for severe educational difficulties include the following.

Developmental problems
- Learning difficulties
- ADHD
- Hearing or visual deficit
- Dyslexia
- Dyspraxia
- ► Autistic spectrum disorder

Social problems
- Family problems at home
- ► Emotional, physical, sexual abuse or neglect
- Peer problems
- Absence from school

School failure is associated with low self-esteem, behavioural difficulties, psychosomatic disorders and has profound effects on adult life. It is important to resolve the problems as early as possible.

Dyslexia
Dyslexia is the most common type of specific learning difficulty. The dyslexic child is unable to process effectively the information required in order to read. The result is a reading ability below that expected for the child's level of intelligence. Children may struggle with spelling and handwriting.

There may be a history of early language delay. If this is unrecognized the child is likely to fail at school, and may respond by withdrawing or disruptive behaviour. The diagnosis should be confirmed by an educational psychologist, and individual help is required to overcome the difficulties. Strategies to help children with dyslexia include allowing extra time to complete written tasks, use of computers as writing aids and adapting the presentation of information to suit their learning style.

Dyspraxia
Motor incoordination leads to significant problems with handwriting, and difficulty with sports and with practical tasks such as dressing and eating with cutlery. If it is disproportionate to their general developmental ability the term 'dyspraxia' or 'developmental coordination disorder' may be applied. The academic and social difficulties that ensue can cause unhappiness and behaviour problems. Occupational therapists have experience in assessing the level of difficulties and can assist in devising therapy programmes, sometimes using equipment to reduce the functional difficulties.

Who is involved?

Health visitors are nurses specially trained in child care and development, and are responsible for most of the Healthy Child Programme. They work in teams, and run child health clinics, visit at home and provide support particularly for families identified as being in need or at risk

School nurses are specially trained to work with children at school. They are responsible for identifying children with medical needs, facilitating their care at school, liaising between professionals and providing general advice to schools on health. They review every child at school entry

General practitioners now have responsibility for the routine aspects of the preschool child health programme, i.e. routine examinations and immunizations

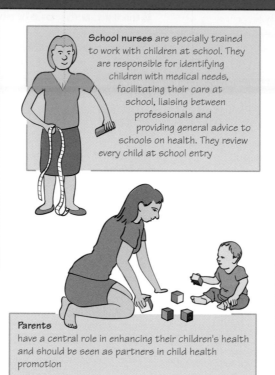

Parents have a central role in enhancing their children's health and should be seen as partners in child health promotion

Community paediatricians specialize in working in the community, including overseeing child health promotion programmes. Some are specialists in child protection, disability or audiology

---

What does the child health promotion involve?

- Guidance in areas of child health

- Health promotion and education

- Prevention of disease by immunization

- Measurement and recording of physical growth

- Monitoring of developmental progress

- Detection of abnormalities

- Identification of children in need

- **Parent-held child health record (the Red Book)**
  Parents are issued with a child health record at their child's birth. It records child health checks; immunizations; the growth chart; parental observations; primary care, dental and hospital visits; and health education and advice
- **Professional records**
  Professionals keep their own record of contact. Computer-based systems are increasingly used, particularly for child health surveillance
- **Special registers**
  Under the Children Act 1989 all social service departments are required to keep registers of children with special needs or chronic illness. They are useful for providing parents with information about services, keeping track of referral and review, anticipating needs and auditing the service. Parental permission is required before placing a child on a register
- **Child Protection Register**
  Social services departments keep a register of children who have been abused or neglected so that professionals can readily determine if a child or others in the family are known to be at risk

Health education and promotion

Young families are growing up more isolated, without the support of extended families. In the UK health promotion is delivered by health visiting teams through the Healthy Child Programme. The programme involves a package of care that includes guidance, immunization, screening and identification of children with a variety of needs. It is underpinned by a principle of progressive universalism where all children receive a basic service with increased input according to a child's or family's needs, so ensuring that the most vulnerable families are supported. Routine contact takes place in the first two weeks, at 6–8 weeks, 6–12 months and at 2–2½ years, and parents can attend drop in clinics when they choose. Sure Start Children's Centres, a UK government initiative, provide skilled staff and facilities where child health promotion is core to their work.

Parental mental health

Parents' ability to provide a quality home life for their families can be profoundly affected by mental health. An important aspect of child health promotion is to recognize when this is an issue and to guide parents towards receiving appropriate help. Postnatal depression is common and health visitors are alert to identifying it and ensuring support is in place.

Parenting support

Many young parents have had little experience of young children before having a baby, and lack the support of an extended family. An important component of health promotion is supporting parents and helping them develop the skills to cope with the challenges of bringing up children. One way is to offer parents the opportunity to participate in a parenting programme where they are helped to enhance their parenting skills and have the benefit of sharing their concerns with others.

Baby care

Guidance is routinely offered to parents about all aspects of baby care, including clothing, bathing, handling and positioning the baby. Information is also given about normal development, what to expect from the child, how to promote learning and how to recognize developmental difficulties. Advice is given about common medical problems, and how to manage them.

Nutrition

Addressing nutritional issues forms a major part of a health visitor's work. It includes promotion of breast-feeding, advice about weaning, dealing with eating difficulties commonly encountered in toddlers, and education about healthy diets for the entire family. Now that obesity is epidemic in children, an important aspect of child health promotion relates to ensuring that children have a healthy balanced diet and to increasing their physical activity (see Chapter 10).

Child development

Early intervention is important if a child has developmental delay or a developmental disorder. A key aspect of child health promotion involves the early detection of developmental concerns and directing the family to appropriate evaluation and input (see Chapter 3).

Behavioural problems

Behavioural concerns around crying, sleep and temper tantrums are universal. Advice and support in the early stages can avoid them developing into major problems.

Immunization and screening

These important aspects of the child health promotion programme are covered in Chapters 8 and 14.

Passive smoking

Children exposed to passive smoking are at greatly increased risk for respiratory disorders. Avoidance of exposing children to smoke at home is an important health promotion issue.

Injury prevention

Most injuries occur in the home, so education of parents can have an important impact on their prevention. Issues of importance include car seats and belts, road safety and use of cycle helmets, gates on stairs, safety in the kitchen, protection against fire hazards, covering electric sockets, and keeping medicines/poisons out of reach.

Identifying risks and safeguarding children

Raising children is a challenging task and it is made more so when families live in poverty, when parents lack education, where there are mental health problems or there is domestic violence. Where there are concerns that a child might be the victim of neglect, non-accidental injury or emotional or sexual abuse, social care needs to be informed (see Chapter 65). Health visiting teams have a key role in monitoring children who require safeguarding and are particularly well placed for this.

Health promotion in school

School provides an invaluable opportunity to educate the young about healthy living, and, hopefully, the school years are a time when adjustments in lifestyle can be made more easily than later on in life. Issues of particular importance that are addressed are:
- Nutrition
- Physical activity
- Reducing risk factors for obesity
- Drugs and alcohol abuse
- Contraception and safe sex
- Sexually transmitted diseases
- Smoking
- Healthy relationships
- Parenting skills.

Immunization and the diseases it protects against

Immunization and the diseases it protects against

Tetanus
- Given IM in infancy as part of DTaP/IPV/Hib, with boosters preschool and in high school
- *Dirty wounds:* Give tetanus immunoglobulin, with booster if last vaccination was >10 years ago (or full course if not immunized)

MMR
- Live attenuated vaccine against:
  - Measles
  - Mumps
  - Rubella
- The vaccine is a live attenuated virus given at 13 months and at school entry. Children who are severely immunosuppressed should not receive the vaccine, nor pregnant girls. Advice is needed if the child is severely allergic to eggs (the vaccine is grown on chick embryo tissue)
- There is no evidence that it is related to autism and bowel disease
- Side effects :
  - common to have rash and fever 5–10 days later
  - mild mumps 2 weeks later

DTaP/IPV/Hib
- Primary immunization given intramuscularly three times in infancy, and then preschool
- Protects against five diseases:
  - Diphtheria (D)
  - Tetanus (T)
  - Pertussis (aP)
  - Polio (IPV)
  - Haemophilus influenzae type B (Hib)
- Pertussis should not be given in a progressive neurological condition
- Possible side effects within 12–24 hours include:
  - swelling and redness at site
  - fever
  - diarrhoea and/or vomiting
  - papule at injection site lasting a few weeks
  - irritability for 48 hours
  - rarely high fever, febrile convulsions, anaphylaxis

National immunization schedule in the UK

Infant

Birth	Hep B and BCG in at risk infants
2 months	DTaP/ IPV/ Hib + pneumococcal
3 months	DTaP/ IPV/ Hib + MenC (meningococcal C)
4 months	DTaP/ IPV/ Hib + MenC + pneumococcal
12 months	Hib + MenC
13 months	MMR + pneumococcal

Preschool

3–5 years	DTaP/ IPV + MMR

Secondary school

13–18 years	Td (diphtheria, tetanus)/IPV
Girls 12 years	HPV

BCG (bacille Calmette–Guérin)
Protects against tuberculosis. Given to babies living in areas with a high rate of TB or to children whose parents or grandparents were born in a TB high prevalence country
- a live attenuated bacterium strain of Mycobacterium bovis
- given intradermally
- papule forms and often ulcerates
- heals over 6–8 weeks with a scar

MenC
Given IM. Protects against infection by meningococcal group C bacteria—meningitis and septicaemia. It does not protect against any other form of meningitis

Pneumoccoccal
Given IM. Protects against pneumococcal infection—pneumonia, septicaemia and meningitis

HPV (human papillomavirus virus)
Protects against common causes of cervical cancer, but not against other sexually transmitted diseases

General immunization guidelines
- immunizations should not be given to a child who:
  - is younger than indicated in the schedule
  - is acutely unwell with fever
  - has had an anaphylactic reaction to a previous dose of the vaccine
- Repeat immunizations should not be given sooner than indicated in the schedule
- If a child misses an immunization, it should be given later. There is no need to restart the course
- Live attenuated vaccines (e.g. measles, mumps, rubella, BCG) should not usually be given to children with immunodeficient states (e.g. cytotoxic therapy or high dose steroids)

In the UK we immunize against the following diseases.

Diphtheria

Diphtheria is now very rare in developed countries. It is caused by the organism *Corynebacterium diphtheriae*. Infection occurs in the throat, forming a pharyngeal exudate, which leads to membrane formation and obstruction of the upper airways. An exotoxin released by the bacterium may cause myocarditis and neuritis with paralysis.

Tetanus

Tetanus is caused by an anaerobic organism, *Clostridium tetani*, found universally in the soil, which enters the body through open wounds. Progressive painful muscle spasms are caused by a neurotoxin produced by the organism. Involvement of the respiratory muscles results in asphyxia and death.

►Pertussis (whooping cough)

Whooping cough is caused by the bacterium *Bordetella pertussis*. It lasts for 6–8 weeks, and has three stages: catarrhal, paroxysmal and convalescent. Paroxysms of coughing are followed by a whoop (a sudden inspiratory effort against a narrowed glottis), with vomiting, dyspnoea and sometimes seizures. Complications include bronchopneumonia, convulsions, apnoea and bronchiectasis. The diagnosis is clinical, and can be confirmed by nasopharyngeal culture. Erythromycin given early shortens the illness, but is ineffective by the time the whoop is heard. There is high morbidity and mortality in children under the age of 2 years.

Polio

Polio is caused by the poliomyelitis virus, which produces a mild febrile illness, progressing to meningitis in some children. Anterior horn cell damage leads to paralysis, pain and tenderness. It may also cause respiratory failure and bulbar paralysis. Residual paralysis is common in those who survive.

Haemophilus influenzae B

Haemophilus influenzae type B (Hib) was the main cause of meningitis (Chapter 14) in young children before the vaccine was introduced. It led to severe neurological sequelae such as profound deafness, cerebral palsy and epilepsy in 10–15% of cases and death in 3%. The vaccine is only effective against type B infection.

Pneumococcal disease

Pneumococcal disease is caused by *Streptococcus pneumoniae*, which can produce serious invasive disease including septicaemia, meningitis and pneumonia.

►Meningococcal C

Meningococcus C causes purulent meningitis in young children with a purpuric rash and septicaemic shock. Mortality is as high as 10% and morbidity includes hearing loss, seizures, brain damage, organ failure and tissue necrosis.

►Measles

Measles is characterized by a maculopapular rash, fever, coryza, cough and conjunctivitis. Complications include encephalitis leading to neurological damage and a high mortality rate. In the UK there has been a recent reduction in vaccine uptake due to unfounded concerns about an association with autism and inflammatory bowel disease. These have now been disproven, but unfortunately there has been an associated increase in cases of measles.

Mumps

Mumps causes a febrile illness with enlargement of the parotid glands. Complications include aseptic meningitis, sensorineural deafness and orchitis in adults. It is a possible cause of subfertility in men.

Rubella

Rubella is a mild illness causing rash and fever. Its importance lies in the devastating effects it has on the fetus if infection occurs in the early stages of pregnancy. These include multiple congenital defects such as cataracts, deafness and congenital heart disease.

►Tuberculosis

Tuberculosis (TB) remains a major problem in many countries and is re-emerging in eastern Europe. It affects the lungs, meninges, bones and joints. Most children with TB are identified because they are contacts of infected adults. Symptoms include cough, tiredness, weight loss, night sweats, haemoptysis and lymphadenopathy. Most individuals with TB have a positive reaction on Mantoux skin testing. Active TB requires treatment that must be continued over many months. Drug-resistant strains are now emerging. BCG is recommended at birth for babies born in communities where there is a high prevalence.

►Hepatitis B

Hepatitis B is an important cause of acute and chronic liver disease. It can be transmitted perinatally from carrier mothers or through blood transfusion, needlestick injuries and biting insects. Children with HBV may be asymptomatic. Babies born to HBsAg +ve mothers receive vaccination at birth.

Human papillomavirus

Infection with human papillomavirus (HPV) is common, with over 50% of sexually active women infected over the course of their lifetime. Two strains of HPV (16 and 18) are the cause of cervical cancer in over 70% of cases.

Weight faltering

(Note that babies may normally cross centiles in the first year)

► Environmental/psychosocial (non-organic)
- Most common cause of weight faltering
- Weight is usually affected first, then height and head growth
- Eating difficulties are common
- Disturbed maternal–infant interaction may be present
- Maternal depression/psychiatric disorder may be present
- Neglect may be a factor

► Cystic fibrosis
(see Chapter 27)
- Diarrhoea
- Chest infections

IUGR
- Low birthweight
- If birth length and head size were also small, catch-up is less likely
- May have features of TORCH
- May be due to a genetic syndrome

Immunodeficiency (rare)
- Recurrent infections
- HIV, SCID are causes

Genetic syndromes
- Low birthweight common
- Dysmorphic features

Chronic illness
- Only rarely an occult cause
- Features depend on the illness

► Gastro-oesophageal reflux
(see Chapter)
- Pain from oesophagitis
- Apnoea
- Vomiting/possetting
- Common in babies with neuro-developmental problems

Coeliac disease (see Chapter)
- Weight may fall off at weaning when gluten is introduced
- Diarrhoea
- Irritability

Endocrine dysfunction
- Developmental delay in hypothyroidism
- Growth hormone deficiency very rare

What you need from your evaluation

History

- **Nutritional history.** Take a dietary history (a food diary can be helpful).
  Ask about feeding difficulties: did they start at birth, weaning or as a toddler? Consider whether they are a result or cause of weight faltering
- **Review of symptoms.** A good history identifies most organic conditions. Look for diarrhoea, colic, vomiting, irritability, fatigue or chronic cough
- **Developmental history.** Are there neurodevelopmental problems? Has weight faltering affected the baby's developmental progress?
- **Past medical history.** Low birthweight and prenatal problems may jeopardize growth potential. Recurrent or chronic illness may affect growth
- **Family history.** Is there a family history of weight faltering or genetic problems? Are there psychosocial problems?

Examination

- **General observations.** Does the child look neglected, ill or malnourished (thin, wasted buttocks, a protuberant abdomen and sparse hair)? How does the mother relate to the baby?
- **Growth.** Plot growth on a chart (remember to correct for prematurity!)
- **Physical examination.** Look for signs of chronic illness

Investigations

'Fishing' for a diagnosis by carrying out multiple investigations is futile. Obtaining a blood count and ferritin level is useful as iron deficiency is common and affects development and appetite. Otherwise, investigations should be based on clinical findings

Concern about growth is usually raised when:
• Weight is below the 2nd centile
• Height is below the 2nd centile
• *Or* when height or weight cross down two centiles.

Growth and weight faltering are common in the first 2 years of life, and expertise is needed to diagnose a normal growth pattern from a pathological cause. There is some debate about the terms used. *Weight faltering* has replaced *failure to thrive* and tends to imply that the condition is not serious and is transient. *Failure to thrive (FTT)* implies not only growth failure, but also failure of emotional and developmental progress. It usually refers to babies or toddlers who have been subject to neglect. The most common causes of weight faltering and failure to thrive are non-organic.

It can be very distressing when a young child's weight falters, and the evaluation needs to be carried out sensitively. The purpose is to differentiate the child with a problem, and to identify contributing factors whether organic or non-organic (which may coexist). It is important that a normal, healthy but small baby is not wrongly labelled as having a problem. Investigations need to be requested judiciously.

▶ Weight faltering due to environmental or psychosocial causes

Psychosocial problems are the commonest cause. Problems may include eating difficulties, difficulties in the home, limitations in the parents, disturbed attachment between mother and child, and maternal depression or psychiatric disorder. Uncommonly, neglect is a factor.

Most commonly the child is from a caring home, where parents are anxious and concerned. The problem is often one of eating difficulties, where meals are very stressful and parents do their utmost (often counter-productively) to persuade the child to eat. The picture is quite different from the neglected child who shows physical signs of poor care and emotional attachment. In this case the problem is often denied and compliance with intervention poor.

Management must suit the underlying problem. An organic cause needs to be excluded first. The family health visitor should then be involved for nutritional advice and help with eating problems. Practical support can ease the stress, and nursery placement can be very helpful as well as helping to resolve eating difficulties. Occasionally it is necessary to admit the baby to hospital for observation.

Failure to thrive

FTT implies not only growth failure, but also failure of emotional and developmental progress. Weight gain is usually first affected, followed in some by a fall in length and head circumference. The child's development may also be delayed. Where neglect is the cause and the family is not amenable to help, social care must be involved. A minority of children need to be removed from their homes.

Malabsorption

Malabsorption is an important cause of poor weight gain. Diarrhoea and colic are usually present as diagnostic clues. The commonest causes of malabsorption are coeliac disease and cystic fibrosis. In the former, the growth curve characteristically shows fall-off in weight coincident with the introduction of gluten to the diet.

Chronic illness

Children and babies with any chronic illness may grow poorly. They rarely present as a diagnostic dilemma as the manifestations of the disease are usually evident. However, organic causes may be compounded by psychosocial difficulties and these need to be addressed. Very rarely, chronic disease can be occult and present as weight faltering. In some cases gastrostomy placement may be required.

Familial causes

Small parents tend to have small children and small, healthy, normal children with short parents should not arouse concern. Usually growth is steady along the lower centiles, but large babies born to small parents may cross down centiles before settling onto their destined line.

Familial causes

Genetic syndromes are quite commonly associated with short stature, often with congenital abnormalities or dysmorphic features. Intrauterine growth retardation (IUGR) results from adverse uterine conditions that may affect infant growth. When this occurs early in gestation, length and head circumference as well as weight may be affected, and growth potential may be jeopardized. The cause of the IUGR should, where possible, be identified.

KEY POINTS

• Be sensitive. It can be very distressing to parents if a baby has weight faltering or fails to thrive.
• Differentiate significant weight faltering from the normal baby who is 'catching down' centiles.
• Identify any symptoms and signs suggestive of organic conditions.
• Only perform laboratory investigations if there are clinical leads in the history and physical examination.
• Identify psychosocial problems that are affecting the baby's growth and provide appropriate help and support.

Steady growth below centiles

▶ Constitutional (familial) short stature
- Short parents
- Normal history and examination
- No delay in bone age

▶ Maturational delay
- Delayed onset of puberty
- Family history of delay
- Delayed bone age

Turner's syndrome
- Features of Turner's syndrome (not always present)
- XO karyotype
- No pubertal signs
- No delay in bone age

IUGR
- Low birthweight
- The underlying reason for the IUGR may be evident

Skeletal dysplasias (rare)
- Body disproportion with shortened limbs
- Achondroplasia is the most common form

Fall-off in growth across centiles

Chronic illness
- Usually identifiable on history and physical examination
- Crohn's disease and chronic renal failure may be occult
- Some delay in bone age occurs

Acquired hypothyroidism
- Clinical features of hypothyroidism
- Goitre may be present
- Low T4, high TSH and thyroid antibodies
- Delayed bone age

Cushing's disease (rare)
- Usually iatrogenic due to prescribed steroids
- Cushingoid features
- Delayed bone age

▶ Growth hormone deficiency (rare)
- Congenital or acquired
- May occur with other hormone deficiencies
- Delayed bone age

Psychosocial
- Neglected appearance
- Behavioural problems
- Catch-up growth occurs when child is removed from home

What you need from your evaluation

History

- **Medical history and review of systems.** Identify any chronic condition, such as asthma, arthritis or diabetes, that can affect growth. Ask about symptoms of raised intracranial pressure, malabsorption and hypothyroidism. Long-term steroid administration stunts growth
- **Family history.** Compare the child's growth with parental heights. It normally lies on the centile between parents' height centiles. Late maternal menarche suggests familial maturational delay
- **Birth history.** A child born small for gestational age may have reduced growth potential. Enquire too about perinatal problems
- **Psychosocial history.** Emotional neglect and abuse can stunt growth but also ascertain whether there are social or emotional difficulties resulting from short stature

Physical examination

- **Pattern of growth.** Obtain previous growth measurements from the GP or school nurse. A fall-off in growth suggests a medical condition requiring treatment
- **Anthropometric measures.** Obtain accurate measures of length (to 24 months of age) or height, and weight. Plot on a growth chart
- **General examination.** Look for signs of hypothyroidism, body disproportion, stigmata of Turner's syndrome and dysmorphism. Each organ system should be examined for evidence of occult disease
- **Head circumference**

Investigations and their significance

If a decrease in growth velocity has occurred, investigations are always required.

Blood count and plasma viscosity	Inflammatory bowel disease
Urea and electrolytes	Chronic renal failure
Coeliac antibodies	Screening test for coeliac disease
Thyroxine and TSH	Hypothyroidism
Karyotype (in girls)	Turner's syndrome
Growth hormone tests	Hypopituitarism, growth hormone deficiency
X-ray of the wrist for bone age	Delayed bone age suggests maturational delay, hypothyroidism, GH deficiency or corticosteroid excess. A prediction of adult height can be made from it

Short stature is usually physiological, and is due to reduced genetic potential or maturational delay (slow physical development). Fall-off in growth is much more concerning as it suggests a pathological cause. Short stature can cause social difficulties, particularly for adolescent boys, and occasionally psychological counselling is required.

Constitutional or familial short stature

Short parents tend to have short children. In this case the history and physical examination are normal, and the bone age appropriate for age. Reassurance is often all that is needed. Prescribing growth hormone in children with physiological short stature is controversial and probably has little effect on the child's final adult height.

Maturational delay

Children with maturational delay are often called 'late developers' or 'late bloomers'. These children are short and reach puberty late. Their final height depends on their genetic constitution, and may be normal. There is often a family history of delayed puberty and menarche, and the bone age is delayed. Most families simply require reassurance that final height will not be so affected. Sometimes, teenage boys find the social pressures are so great that it is helpful to trigger puberty early using low doses of testosterone, so causing an early growth spurt. This treatment does not have an effect on final height.

Hypothyroidism

The most common causes of hypothyroidism are Hashimoto's autoimmune thyroiditis, which is more common in girls, and hypothyroidism secondary to hypopituitarism. A lack of thyroid hormone has a profound effect on growth, and short stature is often the presenting sign. Other features include a fall-off in school performance, constipation, dry skin and delayed puberty. Low thyroxine (T4) and high thyroid stimulating hormone (TSH) levels are found on investigation, along with antithyroid antibodies if the cause is autoimmune. Treatment with thyroid hormone is lifelong. Parents are often alarmed when their placid, hypothyroid child is transformed into a normal, active teenager. The prognosis is good.

Rarer hormonal problems

Cushing's syndrome and disease are extremely rare in childhood. However, growth suppression from exogenous steroids (e.g. high-dose inhaled steroids for asthma) is not uncommon. When children require long-term high-dose oral steroid therapy, the deleterious effect on growth is reduced by giving steroids on alternate days.

Growth hormone deficiency is a rare cause of short stature. It may be idiopathic or may occur secondary to pituitary tumours or cranial irradiation. It may be accompanied by deficiency of other pituitary hormones. The diagnosis is made by growth hormone testing, and brain imaging is needed to identify any underlying pathology. Treatment involves daily subcutaneous injections of synthetic growth hormone.

Chronic illness

Any chronic illness can cause stunting of growth. However, chronic illnesses rarely present as short stature as the features of the illness are usually all too evident. Chronic conditions that present with poor growth before other clinical features become obvious include inflammatory bowel disease, coeliac disease and chronic renal failure.

Turner's syndrome

Turner's syndrome or gonadal dysgenesis is an important cause of short stature and delayed puberty in girls. It is caused by the absence of one X chromosome, although mosaicism also occurs. The gonads are merely streaks of fibrous tissue.

At birth, Turner babies often have webbing of the neck and lymphoedematous hands and feet. In childhood, short stature is marked and girls often have the classic features of webbing of the neck, shield-shaped chest, wide-spaced nipples and a wide carrying angle. Some girls are only diagnosed in adolescence when puberty fails to occur. Growth can be promoted by small doses of growth hormone and oestrogen in childhood. Puberty has to be initiated and maintained by oestrogen therapy. Despite treatment, women with Turner's syndrome are usually short. As a result of recent advances in infertility treatment, a few women have become pregnant through in-vitro fertilization (IVF) with donated ova.

KEY POINTS

• A good history and physical examination identify most pathological causes of short stature.
• Focus on looking for signs of intracranial pathology, hormone deficiency, chronic illness and gastrointestinal symptoms.
• Relate the child's height to the parents' heights.
• Identify any emotional and social consequences of being short.

Causes of obesity

► **Nutritional obesity**
- Family history of obesity is common
- Social/emotional difficulties
- Early puberty
- Boys' genitalia may seem small
- Child tends to be tall

► **Endocrine causes (very rare)**
- Hypothyroidism
- Cushing's
- Hypothalamic lesions

► **Genetic syndromes and single gene defects (rare)**
- Severe obesity from infancy
- Short stature
- Dysmorphic features
- Learning disability
- Hypogonadism
- Other congenital abnormalities

Consequences for obese children
- Low self-esteem
- School problems (bullied and bullies)
- Orthopaedic
- Asthma
- Sleep apnoea
- Polycystic ovary syndrome
- Impaired glucose tolerance
- Hypertension
- Dyslipidaemia
- Abnormal liver function tests

What you need from your evaluation

History

- **Lifestyle and diet.** Ask about both physical activity and sedentary activities. Take a dietary history, but bear in mind this may be a sensitive issue
- **Emotional and behavioural problems.** Social and school problems are very common. Children may be depressed, bullied or be bullies
- **Complications.** Musculoskeletal symptoms occur due to increased load on the joints. Snoring, and lethargy or tiredness during the day are signs of sleep apnoea. Diabetes and cardiovascular disease are rare in childhood (but biochemical indicators are common)
- **Learning difficulties.** Children with an obesity-related genetic syndrome have special educational needs
- **Symptoms** of endocrine causes, but hypothyroidism and Cushing's are rare
- **Family history.** Ask about others who are obese, and early-onset type 2 diabetes and heart disease

Investigations

Investigate for a cause if the child is short, dysmorphic or has learning difficulties
Look for co-morbidity if very obese

Looking for a cause:
- T4, TSH — Low T4 / high TSH in hypothyroidism
- Urinary free cortisol — High in Cushing's disease
- Karyotype and DNA analysis — Genetic syndrome, e.g. Prader–Willi syndrome
- MRI of the brain — Hypothalamic cause

Looking for consequences of obesity:
- Urinary glucose, oral glucose tolerance test — Diabetes
- Fasting lipid screen — Dyslipidaemia
- Liver function tests — Fatty liver

Examination

- **Growth.** Nutritionally obese children are tall. Short stature or fall-off in height suggests a pathological cause. Calculate body mass index (BMI) and plot on a chart
- **Endocrinological signs.** In poor growth look for signs of hypothyroidism (goitre, developmental delay, slow tendon reflexes, bradycardia) and steroid excess (moon face, buffalo hump, striae, hypertension, bruising)
- **Signs of dysmorphic syndromes.** Short stature, microcephaly, hypogonadism, hypotonia and congenital anomalies
- **Signs of complications.** Check blood pressure and look for acanthosis nigricans (a dark velvety appearance at the neck and axillae)—a sign of insulin resistance

Obesity is an increasing problem in childhood and 1 in 10 children are obese even by the time they start primary school. Most overweight and obese children have nutritional obesity, and the diagnosis can be made clinically, as rare causes are accompanied by poor growth and other clinical features such as learning disability and dysmorphic features. In the UK overweight is defined as a body mass index (BMI) above the 91st centile and obesity as BMI above the 98th centile.

At one time obesity in childhood was thought to be a cosmetic problem, but it is now clear that comorbidity can occur in children and adolescents too. The mainstay of management is lifestyle change. Lipase inhibitors to induce fat malabsorption and bariatric surgery are occasionally considered in adolescents.

Nutritional obesity

The metabolic factors that predispose some individuals to becoming obese have yet to be determined and the correlation between nutrient intake and development of obesity is not simple. Nutritionally obese children are tall, but as they tend to develop puberty early, their final adult height is not necessarily tall. Despite its prevalence, obesity remains a stigma and obese children have a high incidence of emotional and behavioural difficulties.

Lifestyle change is difficult to achieve and it is now well recognized that traditional dietary advice that focuses on the child is not effective. Guidance needs to be holistic, family focused and delivered in a skilled way that builds motivation. It includes the following.
• **Support.** Obese children are often the victims of teasing by peers and psychological disturbance is common. Even if weight control is not successful, continuous support is necessary to help these children cope with their condition.
• **Encouraging physical activity and reducing sedentary behaviour.** This may be difficult if obese children experience ridicule when trying to be active.
• **A balanced healthy diet.** Rapid decreases in weight through 'crash dieting' should not be attempted and, while the child is growing, weight maintenance is a reasonable goal.
• **Monitoring** of comorbidity and management when needed.
• Medication and surgery are generally not appropriate or licensed (although may be considered in older adolescents with comorbidity).

Most obese children can be managed in primary care or the community, although those with complex difficulties should be under the care of a paediatrician and multidisciplinary team. Group programmes providing lifestyle education and opportunities for physical activity are increasingly available.

Despite medical intervention, reduction of obesity once it is well established is difficult. Psychological difficulties may well persist into the adult years. Society deals harshly with the obese and studies show that obesity is a handicap later in life. In childhood overt medical complications are few, although metabolic markers for cardiovascular disease, diabetes and fatty liver are common. Obese children are more susceptible to musculoskeletal strain and slipped capital femoral epiphyses. Rarely, insulin-resistant diabetes mellitus develops in childhood. As obese adults, the morbidity is significant with diabetes and hypertension common, leading to early mortality from ischaemic heart disease and strokes. Gallstones and certain cancers are also more prevalent.

Infant obesity

Excessive weight gain and obesity in infancy are now recognized as being far from benign. Epidemiological studies show that this can track into childhood and on to adult life. When obesity in the early years is extreme, genetic syndromes should be considered, particularly when there is dysmorphism, developmental delay and congenital abnormalities. Health visiting teams are beginning to recognize and address excessive weight gain as a problem as concerning as weight faltering.

Public health issues

Prevention

As in most conditions, prevention is better than cure. There is some evidence that breast-feeding in infancy is protective, and promotion of good nutrition in the early years, when food habits are developing, is important. Physical activity needs to be encouraged in all children, not simply the obese. There is a need for these health issues to be addressed in baby clinics and in school, particularly during adolescence when a high intake of high fat foods and decrease in exercise is common. If intervention is provided early in the course of obesity, weight control is likely to be more successful.

Monitoring of obesity

In the UK the National Child Measurement Programme measures children at entry to primary school (age 4–5 years) and on leaving primary school (age 10–11 years). Parents are notified if their child is overweight or obese.

KEY POINTS

• Most obese children have nutritional obesity.
• Emotional and behavioural problems are common.
• There is a high risk of adult obesity and comorbidity.
• Lifestyle management focusing on physical activity and diet is required.
• Rare causes of obesity are associated with poor growth.

Insulin-dependent diabetes mellitus (type 1 diabetes)

Aetiology
- 1 in 500 (0–14 years)
- Destruction of beta islet cells in pancreas leads to insulin deficiency
- Onset determined by genetic predisposition plus some trigger factor (possibly viral infection related)
- Incidence is increasing, particularly in children <5years old

Initial presentation
- Polyuria, polydipsia and weight loss over a few weeks
- Diagnosis if random blood sugar >11.1 mmol/L although transient hyperglycaemia can occasionally be seen without diabetes

Poor diabetic control
- Recurrent admissions with ketoacidosis
- Recurrent severe hypoglycaemia
- Poor growth
- Hyperglycaemia, high HbA1c
- Lipodystrophy if inadequate rotation of injection sites

Hypoglycaemia
- The result of excess insulin or inadequate carbohydrate intake, especially after exercise
- Feel hungry and shaky
- Pale, sweating, tremors
- Tachycardic
- Drowsy or irritable
- Convulsions or coma
- Hypoglycaemia on testing
- May get rebound hyperglycaemia afterwards
- Urgent treatment with 20 g rapid absorbed carbohydrate (2 dextrose tablets or 100 mL high sugar drink)

Diabetic ketoacidosis (DKA)
- May be triggered by infection or poor compliance
- Thirst and polyuria
- Vomiting
- Abdominal pain
- Acetone smell on the breath
- High blood glucose level, ketones in blood and urine
- Metabolic acidosis on blood gas
  - Severe acidosis pH<7.25 needs intravenous insulin and fluids
- Urea raised, electrolytes disturbed
- Signs of dehydration
- Kussmaul acidotic breathing
- Hypovolaemic shock, drowsiness and coma if not treated urgently
- Recurrent DKA suggests major difficulty with self-management and support—needs combined psychological support and medical intervention

Ongoing management
- Requires multidisciplinary approach
- Initial correction of metabolic state and education of family
- Treatment with insulin and specific dietary advice
- Monitoring blood sugar levels at home and HbA1c regularly in clinic
- Education about diabetic control, injection technique, diet and exercise
- Dealing with emergencies and liaison with school

Prognosis
- Retinopathy, neuropathy, renal impairment and atherosclerosis are the long-term effects of poor control of blood glucose levels

What you need from your evaluation

History
- Ask about polyuria, polydipsia, lethargy and weight loss
- Ask about bedwetting (secondary enuresis)
- Review the diabetic diary and ask about hypoglycaemic and hyperglycaemic episodes—what triggered them and were they managed appropriately?
- How is the child coping at home and at school? Also ask about siblings
- Is the child managing to eat a healthy diet and modify the diet to certain situations (e.g. snacks before heavy exercise)
- Is insulin being administered correctly with rotation of injection sites?

Examination
- Monitor height and weight as poor growth reflects poor control
- Check for signs of lipodystrophy or lipoatrophy at injection sites
- Check blood pressure annually and fundi in older children (>14 years)
- Check for signs of coexistent coeliac disease or hypothyroidism

Investigations and their significance

Blood glucose	Monitor regularly at home using finger-prick samples and handheld glucometer
HbA1c (% of glycosylated haemoglobin)	Reflects control over last 2–3 months
Urinalysis	For glycosuria, ketones, microalbuminuria
Blood gases, U&E	Need to be monitored carefully during acute diabetic ketoacidosis
Coeliac screen	Screen for coeliac disease with antitissue transglutaminase (tTG) or anti-endomysial antibodies
Thyroid function tests and antithyroid antibody screen	Screen for hypothyroidism
Glucose tolerance test (GTT)	In type 2 diabetes
Triglycerides and cholesterol	
Annual retinal screening (>12 years of age)	
Islet cell antibodies, insulin antibodies, GAD antibodies	To confirm autoimmune process at diagnosis
Insulin and C-Peptide levels	Helps distinguish type 1 from type 2 diabetes

Diabetes mellitus

Diabetes affects 1 in 400–500 children and adolescents. It is defined as persistent hyperglycaemia (fasting blood glucose >7 mmol/L). The diagnosis has a major impact on the child and the family in terms of their daily life; the risk of serious illness such as diabetic ketoacidosis (DKA) and the risk of long-term complications such as retinopathy, renal failure, cardiovascular disease and neuropathy.

Type 1 diabetes mellitus

Diabetes in children is usually insulin-dependent diabetes mellitus (type 1) due to autoimmune destruction of the beta cells in the islets of Langerhans in the pancreas, resulting in a lack of insulin. The lack of insulin means that glucose cannot be utilized, resulting in hyperglycaemia. The high glucose concentration in the blood spills over into the urine, causing an osmotic diuresis with polyuria and dehydration. This leads to excessive thirst, and weight loss. Because the cells cannot utilize glucose they switch to metabolizing fats, leading to the production of ketones, resulting in acidosis.

Type 2 diabetes mellitus

In this form of diabetes the pancreas is able to secrete insulin but there is peripheral insulin resistance. Until recently type 2 diabetes was rare in childhood, but the incidence is increasing, probably related to increased calorie intake and reduced exercise. Management is dietary control of carbohydrate and oral hypoglycaemic agents (e.g. sulphonylureas). In some cases the need to produce high levels of insulin leads the pancreas to 'burn out', such that insulin therapy becomes necessary.

Other types of diabetes mellitus

It is increasingly recognized that there are genetic forms of non-insulin-dependent diabetes mellitus which present in childhood. They are often due to impaired secretion of insulin from the pancreatic beta cells. In other cases the diabetes is caused by drugs (e.g. corticosteroids following transplantation) or by disease processes (e.g. cystic fibrosis or pancreatitis) or is associated with genetic syndromes.

Initial presentation of type 1 diabetes

Children usually present with a short (2–3 week) history of lethargy, weight loss, polyuria and thirst. The polyuria may cause a recurrence of bedwetting. If the symptoms are not recognized the child may develop signs of diabetic ketoacidosis with abdominal pain, vomiting and eventually coma. Newly diagnosed children who are ketoacidotic will need admission to hospital to correct dehydration and commence intravenous insulin.

Intensive education of the child and family is needed undertaken by diabetic nurse specialist, paediatric diabetologist and specialist dietician. The child and family are taught how to inject the insulin, monitor blood glucose, test for ketones, and recognize the signs of hypoglycaemia. Children are encouraged to wear a Medic-Alert bracelet, giving details of their condition in case of sudden hypoglycaemic collapse. Education should be structured so that every child has access to the full support available and their progress in building expert knowledge can be verified.

Growing up with diabetes

The education given to families at the time of diagnosis is crucial in developing the right approach to their child's diabetes. As the child gets older they can gradually take on more of the responsibility themselves, including injecting insulin and monitoring blood glucose levels. Normal healthy diet should be encouraged to ease blood sugar regulation.

Managing any chronic condition places an added difficulty on emotional well-being particularly through times when it is normal to show rebellious defiant behaviour such as at adolescence. Diabetes increases the risk of psychological problems (such as eating disorder) linked to poor compliance. The diabetes team need specialist skills in engaging and motivational interviewing of adolescents to help manage these problems.

Insulin therapy (type 1 diabetes)

Many children go through a 'honeymoon' period soon after diagnosis where they need very little insulin, as they still produce some endogenous insulin. More insulin is often required as they go through the pubertal growth spurt. Insulin is usually delivered by an injection pen. Various insulin regimens are used.

• **Twice daily regimen**: the insulin is given as a mixture of rapid-acting insulin (peak at 2–4 hours) and intermediate-acting isophane insulin (peak at 4–12 hours). This is administered subcutaneously in the arms, thighs, buttocks or abdomen, before breakfast and before the evening meal.

• **Basal bolus regimen**: this provides a long-acting insulin at night and rapid-acting insulin given before each meal, based on the calculated carbohydrate intake.

An alternative to these regimens is **continuous subcutaneous insulin infusion** (CSII) of rapid acting insulin via a pump, with the ability to increase the rate (bolus) during mealtimes. The insulin is infused through a cannula, which is changed every third day. This system can give better glycaemic control and fewer hypoglycaemic episodes.

Monitoring

Control is assessed by keeping a blood sugar diary and measuring HbA1c levels, which measures glycaemic control in the preceding few months. The family need to be warned of the symptoms of hypoglycaemia (see opposite) and have carbohydrate available (dextrose tablets) at all times. Screening for complications and associated conditions (thyroid disease, coeliac disease) is performed regularly.

KEY POINTS

• Diabetes is very common: it occurs in 1 in 500 children.
• Presentation is with a short history of weight loss, polyuria and polydipsia.
• DKA can be life-threatening and needs high-dependency treatment
• Insulin is given subcutaneously in a number of different regimen to best suit the child.
• Patients must be able to recognize and treat hypoglycaemia.
• Type 2 diabetes is becoming more common in children.

Presentation of congenital heart defects

Presenting with heart failure

▶ Ventricular septal defect (VSD)
- 32% of congenital heart disease (CHD) (most common)
- Membranous or muscular
- Can be asymptomatic
- Harsh pansystolic murmur at lower left sternal edge
- Parasternal thrill
- Heart failure at 4–6 weeks
- Many close spontaneously

Atrioventricular septal defect(AVSD)
- 5% of CHD
- Atrial and ventricular communication
- May have single atrioventricular valve
- Associated with Down's syndrome (40%)
- Superior axis on ECG

▶ Patent ductus arteriosus (PDA)
- 12% of CHD
- Continuous machinery murmur below left clavicle
- Collapsing pulse
- More common in premature infants

Ventricular septal defect

Patent ductus

Presenting with shock

▶ Coarctation of aorta
- 6% of CHD
- If severe, presents as shock when duct closes in first few days of life
- May present with heart failure and a murmur over the back
- Causes hypertension in older children
- Weak or absent femoral pulses
- Associated with Turner's syndrome

Narrowing (coarctation) of the aorta

Aortic valve stenosis
- 5% of CHD
- If severe, presents as shock or heart failure when duct closes
- May present as asymptomatic murmur
- Older children may have syncope or reduced exercise tolerance
- Ejection systolic murmur radiating to neck

Narrowed aortic valve

Presenting with a murmur
(see Chapter 20)

Pulmonary valve stenosis
- 8% of CHD
- If critical stenosis, may be cyanosed at birth and duct dependent
- Ejection systolic murmur in pulmonary area radiating to back
- Evidence of right ventricular hypertrophy on ECG

Atrial septal defect (ASD)
- 6% of CHD
- Ostium secundum (defect of foramen ovale and atrial septum)
- Ostium primum (defect of atrioventricular septum)
- Usually asymptomatic at birth
- Fixed split second heart sound
- Pulmonary flow murmur
- Recurrent chest infections
- Heart failure

Narrowed pulmonary valve

Thickened muscle

Atrial septal defect

Presenting with cyanosis

Tetralogy of Fallot
- 6% of CHD
- Ejection systolic murmur
- Intermittent cyanosis from birth
- Right ventricular hypertrophy on ECG
- Boot-shaped heart and oligaemic lung fields on chest radiograph

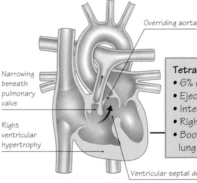

Overriding aorta

Narrowing beneath pulmonary valve

Right ventricular hypertrophy

Ventricular septal defect

▶ Transposition of the great arteries
- 5% of CHD
- Separate pulmonary and systemic circulations, connected only by PDA (or sometimes VSD)
- Severe cyanosis and acidosis at birth
- Requires atrial septostomy urgently followed by definitive 'switch' operation

Aorta

Arterial duct

Connection between the atria

Main pulmonary artery

Investigations and their signficance

Pulse oximetry	To determine degree of cyanosis or check for postductal drop (screening for CHD)
Chest radiograph	Cardiomegaly in heart failure Boot-shaped heart (Fallot's tetralogy) Increased vascular markings with left to right shunts (VSD, ASD, PDA)
ECG	Right ventricular hypertrophy Superior QRS axis (AVSD, primum ASD)
Echo	Ultrasound examination of the heart, usually performed by a paediatric cardiologist, can diagnose the vast majority of congenital heart defects
Fetal echo	Many defects can be detected antenatally
Cardiac catheter	To define complex anatomy or perform non-invasive treatment (e.g. balloon dilatation of stenosed valve)

Congenital heart disease (CHD) is the commonest congenital malformation (7–8 per 1000 livebirths). About 8% are associated with chromosomal abnormality (e.g. AVSD in Down's syndrome) or genetic abnormalities, such as a deletion at chromosome 22q11 which is associated with aortic arch defects and hypocalcaemia (diGeorge syndrome). The risk of CHD is higher if there is a family history. Teratogens may cause CHD (e.g. VSD and tetralogy of Fallot in fetal alcohol syndrome and Ebstein's anomaly after fetal lithium exposure).

Many severe forms of CHD are diagnosed antenatally. Others present at birth, with cyanosis (e.g. transposition of the great arteries or pulmonary atresia) or shock (hypoplastic left heart syndrome). Some duct-dependent lesions present when the arterial duct closes within the first few days (e.g. coarctation of the aorta, severe pulmonary stenosis). Defects with a left to right shunt (e.g. VSD) present with heart failure and difficulty feeding some weeks after birth. Finally, some lesions may be asymptomatic and are first detected as a heart murmur (e.g. ASD, aortic stenosis) (see Chapter 20).

Medical management involves the control of heart failure, pending definitive repair. Many defects can just be monitored for years, and may not need surgical correction.

Congenital heart disease that typically presents in the newborn period

► Coarctation of the aorta

This is a narrowing of the aortic arch. Severe coarctation presents in the first few days of life when the duct closes and insufficient blood is able to reach the lower limbs and perfuse vital organs, causing circulatory collapse and acidosis. The key feature is weak or impalpable femoral pulses. Blood pressure may be higher in the arms than the legs and oxygen saturation will be lower in the feet than the (preductal) right hand. Milder forms of coarctation present with heart failure and a murmur or with hypertension in a young adult. The immediate management is IV prostaglandin E2 to keep the arterial duct patent. Once the diagnosis is confirmed by echocardiography, the narrowed segment is repaired surgically or dilated using a balloon. In girls with Turner's syndrome, 5–10% have coarctation and a proportion may also have a bicuspid aortic valve and aortic dissection in adulthood.

► Transposition of the great arteries

In transposition of the great arteries (TGA), the aorta and main pulmonary artery are transposed, so that the aorta comes off the right ventricle and the pulmonary artery off the left ventricle. TGA always presents soon after birth with profound cyanosis and acidosis. The only way oxygenated blood from the lungs can reach the systemic circulation is across the arterial duct, or a VSD, if present. The emergency management is to commence a prostaglandin infusion, provide ventilatory and circulatory support and perform an atrial septostomy which allows mixing of oxygenated and deoxygenated blood. The definitive treatment is the 'switch' operation, where the two great vessels are switched over and the coronary arteries are reconnected to the new aorta. TGA can be missed on antenatal ultrasound scan since the basic 'four-chamber' view is normal.

Tetralogy of Fallot

Tetralogy of Fallot is the commonest cyanotic defect, representing 6–10% of all CHD. 'Tetralogy' refers to a large VSD, an aorta that sits over the ventricular septum, pulmonary infundibular stenosis and right ventricular hypertrophy. The pulmonary narrowing causes a right-to-left shunt across the VSD. Some present with cyanosis at birth but others are diagnosed by an ejection systolic murmur. Classically these children develop hypercyanotic 'spells' which are relieved by squatting down (to reverse the right-to-left shunt by increasing left ventricular pressure). CXR may show a 'boot-shaped' heart. Surgical correction is usually performed at 2–3 months of age. Tetralogy of Fallot can have a genetic cause and is seen in fetal alcohol syndrome.

► Patent ductus arteriosus

During fetal life the arterial duct shunts blood from the pulmonary artery to the aorta, bypassing the unexpanded lungs. Normally the duct closes within a few days of birth, first by constriction and then by fibrosis. In sick preterm or hypoxic babies it remains open. As the right-sided pressures are now less than the aortic pressure, blood shunts from the systemic to the pulmonary circulation causing cardiac failure and pulmonary oedema. The clinical signs of a patent ductus arteriosus (PDA) are a continuous 'machinery' murmur below the left clavicle and collapsing pulses. A PDA is particularly common in premature infants receiving mechanical ventilation (up to 20%). Management involves diuretics and fluid restriction, and sometimes administration of prostaglandin synthetase inhibitors (e.g. indomethacin or ibuprofen). Rarely the duct needs to be closed by surgical ligation or by a trans-catheter occlusion device.

Causes of heart murmurs in older children

Innocent murmurs
- Have no clinical significance
- Are systolic and musical
- Do not radiate
- Vary with posture and position

Pathological murmurs
- Are pansystolic or diastolic
- Are harsh or long
- May radiate and have a thrill
- Often have associated cardiac symptoms or signs

Venous hum
- Blowing continuous murmur in systole and diastole
- Heard below the clavicles
- Disappears on lying down

Pulmonary flow murmur
- Brief high-pitched murmur at second left intercostal space
- Best heard with child lying down

Systolic ejection murmur
- Short systolic murmur at left sternal edge or apex
- Musical sound
- Changes with child's position
- Intensified by fever, exercise and emotion

► Aortic stenosis
- Soft systolic ejection murmur at right upper sternal border
- Radiates to neck and down left sternal border
- Causes dizziness and loss of consciousness in older children

Atrial septal defect
- Soft systolic murmur at second left intercostal space
- Wide fixed splitting of the second sound
- May not be detected until later childhood

Pulmonary stenosis
- Short systolic ejection murmur in upper left chest
- Conducted to back
- Preceded by ejection click
- Thrill in the pulmonary area

► Ventricular septal defect
- Harsh pansystolic murmur at lower left sternal border
- Radiates all over chest
- Signs of heart failure may be present

► Coarctation of the aorta (see Chapter 19)
- Systolic murmur on left side of chest
- Radiates to the back
- Absent or delayed femoral pulses
- Hypertension

NB: Patent ductus arteriosus and tetralogy of Fallot are discussed in Chapter 19

What you need from your evaluation

History

- Fatigue is the most important symptom of cardiac failure. A baby in cardiac failure can take only small volumes of milk, becomes short of breath on sucking, and becomes sweaty. The older child tires on walking and may become breathless too
- Take a family history. The risk of heart defects is higher in siblings of children with congenital heart disease

Physical examination

- **Murmur.** The quality of the sound and the site where it is heard indicates if it is pathological. Listen for radiation over the precardium, back and neck, with the child both sitting and lying
- **Signs of heart failure:** Look for failure to thrive and poor growth, tachycardia and tachypnoea, crepitations and hepatomegaly (peripheral oedema is rare in children)
- **Pulse and blood pressure:** Remember that femoral pulses are weak, delayed or absent in coarctation of the aorta. Blood pressure will be higher in the arms than the legs
- **Sternal heave:** Indicates right ventricular hypertrophy (e.g. tetralogy of Fallot, pulmonary hypertension)
- **Cyanosis:** An unlikely finding in children presenting with a heart murmur

Investigations and their significance

These are required only if the murmur is thought to be pathological.
- **Echocardiography.** Evaluates cardiac structure and performance, gradients across stenotic valves and the direction of flow across a shunt
- **Chest radiograph.** Provides information about cardiac size and shape, and pulmonary vascularity
- **ECG.** Provides information about ventricular or atrial hypertrophy
- **24 hour ECG.** If associated with symptoms of palpitations or syncope
- **Cardiac catheterization.** Rarely required for diagnosis

Heart murmurs are very common in infants and young children. Most are 'functional' or 'innocent' and are not associated with structural abnormalities. It is important to learn to distinguish these from murmurs associated with cardiac disease. Once a structural lesion has been excluded, the benign nature of the murmur should be discussed with the parents. It is helpful to describe it as a simple 'noise' which itself does not indicate a cardiac defect. Innocent flow murmurs may be more apparent at times of illness or fever.

Defects causing a left-to-right shunt
These are the commonest defects. If large, a considerable volume of blood is shunted, causing hypertrophy, ventricular dilatation and congestive cardiac failure. They usually present as breathlessness. The child is not cyanosed.

▶ Ventricular septal defect (VSD)
This is the commonest congenital lesion. If the VSD is small the child may be asymptomatic but a large shunt causes breathlessness on feeding and crying, poor growth and recurrent chest infections. A harsh, rasping, pansystolic murmur is heard at the lower left sternal border and in large defects the heart is enlarged, a thrill is present and the murmur radiates over the whole chest. There may be signs of heart failure. Loudness of the murmur is not related to the size of the shunt. In large defects cardiomegaly and large pulmonary arteries are seen on the chest radiograph and biventricular hypertrophy on ECG. Echocardiography confirms the diagnosis.

Prevention of endocarditis is important. Small muscular defects usually close spontaneously. Large membranous defects with cardiac failure are initially managed medically, but surgical treatment may be required. If uncorrected, the increased pulmonary blood flow can lead to pulmonary hypertension which eventually leads to reversal of the shunt and intractable cyanosis. (Eisenmenger's syndrome).

Ventricular septal defect

Ventricular septal defect
Large flow causes cardiomegaly and prominent pulmonary arteries

Atrial septal defect (ASD)
As the murmur is soft, it may not be detected until later childhood. The systolic murmur is heard in the second left interspace, and is due to high flow across the normal pulmonary valve and not due to flow across the ASD itself. The second heart sound is widely split and 'fixed' (does not vary with respiration). The child may experience breathlessness, tiredness on exertion or recurrent chest infections. If the defect is moderate or large, closure is carried out either by open heart surgery or using a cardiac catheter. The outcome is usually good. If untreated, cardiac arrhythmias can develop in early adulthood.

Atrial septal defect

Atrial septal defect
High flow through pulmonary valve causes a systolic murmur

Obstructive lesions
Obstructive lesions can occur at the pulmonary and aortic valves and along the aorta. The chamber of the heart proximal to the lesion hypertrophies, and heart failure may develop.

Aortic stenosis
Aortic stenosis is usually identified at routine examination, but some children may experience syncope or dizziness on exertion. The systolic ejection murmur is heard at the right upper sternal border and radiates to the neck. It may be preceded by an ejection click and the aortic second sound is soft and delayed. The peripheral pulse is of small volume and blood pressure may be low. A thrill may be palpable at the lower left sternal border and over the carotid arteries.

Chest radiography may show a prominent left ventricle and ascending aorta. Left ventricular hypertrophy is found on ECG. Echocardiography can evaluate the exact site and severity of the obstruction. Severe stenosis is relieved by balloon valvuloplasty—a catheter is passed from the femoral artery and a balloon inflated to widen the stenosis. If unsuccessful, open heart surgery is required. The Ross procedure involves replacing the damaged aortic valve with the patient's own pulmonary valve, and then fitting a replacement pulmonary valve. Children with aortic stenosis are at risk for sudden death and so this is one defect in which strenuous activity and competitive sports should be avoided.

Narrowed aortic valve

Aortic stenosis
The stenosis causes enlargement of the left ventricle and prominence of the ascending aorta

Pulmonary stenosis
The pulmonary valve is narrowed and the right ventricle hypertrophied. A short ejection systolic murmur is heard over the upper left anterior chest and is conducted to the back. It is usually preceded by an ejection click. With mild stenosis there are usually no symptoms. In severe stenosis a systolic thrill is palpable in the pulmonary area. On chest radiograph dilatation of the pulmonary artery is seen beyond the stenosis, and if severe an enlarged right atrium and ventricle. The extent of the stenosis can be demonstrated by echocardiography and cardiac catheterization. If severe, balloon valvuloplasty is performed. Surgery is generally successful.

Narrowed pulmonary valve

Pulmonary stenosis
Right ventricle hypertrophies to overcome the obstruction

Prophylaxis for infective endocarditis
Any child with significant congenital heart disease is at risk for developing infective endocarditis, particularly if there is a high velocity shunt or abnormal valves. It is important to reduce the risk of bacterial endocarditis by maintaining healthy teeth and gums, but antibiotic prophylaxis for dental or clean surgery is no longer recommended. Body piercing is not advisable.

Causes of acute fever

► Viral infections, e.g.
- Non-specific viral infection
- Upper respiratory tract infection (URTI)

Otitis media
- Tugging at ears, pain
- Red tympanic membrane

Dehydration

Tonsillitis
- Commonly viral
- Sore throat
- Large tonsillar glands
- Smelly breath

Post immunization

Septic arthritis
- Painful joint
- Swelling and effusion

► Serious blood infection, e.g.
- Meningococcal septicaemia
- Streptococcal sepsis
- Toxic shock syndrome
- Malaria

Influenza
- Fever, cough, headache, anorexia
- Arthralgia

Viral illness with rash, e.g.
- Chickenpox
- Measles
- Rubella
- Non-specific viral rash

Pneumonia
- Cough, tachypnoea, retractions
- Signs of consolidation, crackles

Urinary tract infection
(see p. OOO)
- Frequency, dysuria
- Loin or suprapubic pain
- Vomiting
- Abnormal dipstick test and positive microscopy

Post surgery

Kawasaki's disease
- Rash, conjunctivitis, lymphadenopathy, cracked lips, fever, skin peeling

Factitious
- Taking temperature after hot drink
- Deliberate manipulation of thermometer
- Excessive crying or exertion
- Overheating due to swaddling

What you need from your evaluation

History

- Ask about duration and pattern of the fever—does it occur at particular times of the day?
- Is there pain? Earache, difficulty swallowing, dysuria or frequency may point to the source
- Are there associated features such as malaise, anorexia, vomiting, coryza, cough or rash?
- Has there been contact with other infection such as meningitis or chickenpox?
- Has the child just been vaccinated?
- Is the child drinking adequate amounts of fluid?
- What antipyretics and cooling measures have been tried?

Investigations and their significance

- Full blood count — Leucocytosis with neutrophilia suggests bacterial infection
- Throat swab — Streptococcus requires treatment with penicillin
- Blood culture — If positive, suggests septicaemia. Treatment may have to start before result known
- Lumbar puncture — To exclude meningitis and encephalitis. Should be performed in any seriously ill child when no focus of infection can be found, especially in infants <1 year
- Urine analysis — Pure growth of a single organism with significant leucocytosis confirms infection. Protein and red cells may be present. Dipsticks can be used to test for leucocytes, protein and nitrites
- Chest radiograph — May reveal cause of fever in infants as chest signs are not always apparent

Examination

- Check the temperature: oral, axillary or rectal
- Does the child look seriously ill? Is there rash, tachypnoea, tachycardia or dehydration?
- **Chest:** are there signs of respiratory infection—tachypnoea, recession, crackles or grunting?
- **Throat:** feel for cervical lymphadenopathy and look at tonsils. Is there an exudate?
- **Ears:** are the tympanic membranes red or bulging?
- **CNS:** is the child orientated? Is there floppiness or signs of meningism?
- **Urine:** check the urine with dipstick/ microscopy

Fever is usually a response to infection or inflammation and may form part of the body's defence against infection. The height of the fever does not necessarily correlate with the severity of the illness and fever can commonly occur in children with minor illnesses. The child often appears flushed as blood vessels in the skin vasodilate in an attempt to lose heat. Some young children experience febrile convulsions if their temperature rises very rapidly (see Chapter 41).

Temperature can be measured rectally, orally or in the axilla using a thermometer, or using a thermal device in the ear canal or skin. Fever is defined as an axillary temperature above 37°C. It can be treated by undressing the child so heat is lost through the skin. Sponging with tepid water can help. Fever needs treatment with antipyretics such as paracetamol or ibuprofen when it causes discomfort—aspirin should not be used under the age of 12 years as it can lead to severe liver failure (Reye's syndrome, see Chapter 48). Persistent or recurrent fever is discussed in Chapter 22.

Fever in young infants

Fever in infants less than 8 weeks old must be taken seriously as signs of sepsis at this age can be non-specific. Significant fever should always prompt a careful examination and investigations. If ill, infants require a full infection screen including urine culture, chest radiograph and possibly lumbar puncture.

▶Viral upper respiratory tract infections

Upper respiratory tract infections (URTIs) are extremely common in children, occurring on average 6–8 times a year. They are especially common when toddlers start nursery and on starting school when children become exposed to a large number of viral infections to which they have no immunity. Symptoms include coryza (runny nose), acute pharyngitis and fever. In acute pharyngitis the tonsillar fauces and palate are inflamed, cervical lymph nodes may be enlarged and the tympanic membranes inflamed. Young infants may have difficulty breathing and feeding because they are obligate nose breathers. Treatment is symptomatic, with antipyretics such as paracetamol. Saline drops may improve nasal congestion in infants. The infection usually lasts 3–4 days. Antibiotics should not be given.

Tonsillitis

Tonsillitis is usually viral in origin. In older children the commonest bacterial organism is group A beta-haemolytic streptococcus. Symptoms include sore throat or dysphagia and usually a fever. There is often tender cervical lymphadenopathy, which may cause neck stiffness, and associated adenitis in the mesenteric nodes may cause abdominal pain. On examination the tonsils are enlarged and acutely inflamed. In bacterial tonsillitis the breath may smell offensive and there may be a white exudate, although this is not always a reliable sign. Exudates can also occur with infectious mononucleosis (glandular fever) and with diphtheria (now very rare). Acute tonsillitis should be distinguished from hypertrophied but non-inflamed tonsils which are common in preschool children.

Most children do not require antibiotics and can be managed with saline gargles/throat lozenges and paracetamol. If bacterial infection is suspected this should ideally be confirmed by a throat swab. Streptococcal tonsillitis should be treated with benzyl penicillin for 10 days.

Complications of tonsillitis are rare and include otitis media, peritonsillar abscess (quinsy) and poststreptococcal glomerulonephritis. Chronically enlarged tonsils can cause upper airway obstruction and obstructive sleep apnoea. This is an indication for tonsillectomy.

Infectious mononucleosis

Glandular fever is due to Epstein–Barr virus (EBV) infection and is usually a self-limiting infection in adolescents. It presents with low-grade fever, malaise, pharyngitis and cervical lymphadenopathy. Occasionally, hepatosplenomagaly and jaundice may occur. Peripheral leucocytosis with atypical lymphocytes and a positive agglutination test (monospot) are diagnostic. Most adults show serological evidence of EBV infection. The symptoms may last many weeks. Amoxicillin is contraindicated as it will cause a maculopapular rash in EBV infection.

Acute otitis media

Otitis media is very common, especially in young children and can occur in babies. The commonest causes are *Streptococcus pneumoniae*, *Haemophilus influenzae* and viruses. It is especially common when there is eustachian tube dysfunction, which occurs as a result of URTIs, obstruction from enlarged adenoids, cleft palate and in Down's syndrome. Symptoms include fever, deafness and pain in the ear. The child may be irritable and pull at the ear, although infection may also be asymptomatic. Examination shows a red, inflamed and bulging tympanic membrane, with loss of the light reflex. Most cases resolve spontaneously and a trial of symptomatic treatment (paracetamol) for 72 hours is recommended before considering antibiotics. Bacterial otitis media is shortened by treatment with amoxicillin. Prognosis is generally good even if the tympanic membrane has perforated.

Complications include conductive deafness, mastoiditis and secretory otitis media (glue ear)—a thick, glue-like exudate in the middle ear. In secretory otitis media the tympanic membrane looks thickened and retracted with an absent light reflex. If there is significant hearing loss, ventilation tubes (grommets) may be inserted through the tympanic membrane to allow the middle ear to drain. They often fall out after a period of months to years and their use is controversial; but they are indicated if there is language delay secondary to conductive deafness due to glue ear.

KEY POINTS

- Fever is very common in children, and can usually be managed by simple cooling and paracetamol.
- Any ill child with high fever must be examined carefully to exclude serious infections such as meningitis, urinary tract infection or pneumonia.
- Fever in babies less than 8 weeks old must be taken seriously.
- Otitis media and tonsillitis are common causes of fever in young children.
- Most fevers are due to non-specific viral infections or URTIs.

Causes of persistent fever

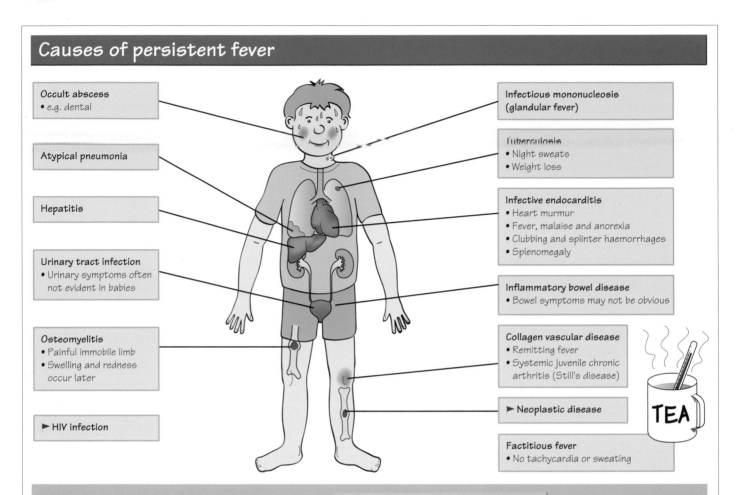

Occult abscess
- e.g. dental

Atypical pneumonia

Hepatitis

Urinary tract infection
- Urinary symptoms often not evident in babies

Osteomyelitis
- Painful immobile limb
- Swelling and redness occur later

▶ **HIV infection**

Infectious mononucleosis (glandular fever)

Tuberculosis
- Night sweats
- Weight loss

Infective endocarditis
- Heart murmur
- Fever, malaise and anorexia
- Clubbing and splinter haemorrhages
- Splenomegaly

Inflammatory bowel disease
- Bowel symptoms may not be obvious

Collagen vascular disease
- Remitting fever
- Systemic juvenile chronic arthritis (Still's disease)

▶ **Neoplastic disease**

Factitious fever
- No tachycardia or sweating

TEA

What you need from your evaluation

History

- Review symptoms related to all organ systems
- Immunization history
- Contact with infectious diseases (e.g. TB)
- Travel history (including visitors)
- Exposure to animals (e.g. tick bites)

Physical examination

(Repeat physical examinations may be required.)

- **Check the temperature chart.** Repetitive chills (rigors) and temperature spikes suggest septicaemia, abscess, pyelonephritis or endocarditis. There is no tachycardia or sweating in factitious fever
- **Examine the mouth and sinuses.** Oral candida may indicate immune deficiency. A red pharynx may suggest infectious mononucleosis. Tap the sinuses and teeth for tenderness
- **Palpate muscles and bones.** Point tenderness suggests osteomyelitis or neoplastic disease. Generalized muscle tenderness occurs in collagen vascular disease. Examine joints carefully for signs of inflammation
- **Heart.** A new murmur or changed murmur may suggest infective endocarditis

Investigations and their significance

● Full blood count	High white cell count in bacterial infection. Very high in leukaemia
● Urinalysis and culture	Occult urinary tract infection
● Examination of blood smear	Parasitic infections, e.g. malaria
● CRP	Raised in infection and inflammation. Trend may be more important than exact level
● ESR or plasma viscosity	High in bacterial infection. Very high in collagen vascular disease, malignancy
● Blood cultures (aerobic and anaerobic)	Bacterial infection. Repeat samples needed to diagnose endocarditis, osteomyelitis and occult abscess
● Liver function tests	Hepatitis
● Mantoux	TB
● Radiographs—chest, bones, sinuses	Characteristic findings with bacterial infection
● Bone marrow aspirate	Leukaemia, metastatic neoplasms, rare infections
● Serological tests	Infectious mononucleosis, other infections, rarely helpful in collagen vascular disease
● Isotope scans	Bone scans or radiolabelled white cell scans may help identify cryptogenic infection such as osteomyelitis or intra-abdominal abscess
● Echocardiography	Vegetations seen on heart valves in endocarditis
● Abdominal ultrasound	Identification of intra-abdominal abscess
● Total body CT or MRI scanning	Detection of neoplasms and abscess

Persistent fever and pyrexia of unknown origin

Pyrexia of unknown origin (PUO) refers to prolonged fever (more than 1 week in young children and 2–3 weeks in adolescents). Often the diagnosis becomes apparent or the fever resolves within a short period of time. The cause is usually an atypical presentation of a common illness such as urine infection or pneumonia, but more significant causes include endocarditis, collagen vascular diseases, malignancy and inflammatory bowel disease. Sometimes no diagnosis is made, but the fever abates spontaneously.

The child should be hospitalized for careful observation. Antipyretics should not be given as they obscure the pattern of fever. Blood cultures should be obtained at the time of fever peaks when the yield is higher.

Kawasaki's disease

Kawasaki's disease should be considered particularly in younger children and in infants with pyrexia beyond five days. Raised inflammatory markers and platelet count are sometimes seen, complications of coronary artery anuerysms.

Infective endocarditis

Infective endocarditis usually occurs as a complication of congenital heart disease. The commonest causal organism is *Streptococcus viridans* which may be introduced during dental or other surgery. Endocarditis can also be seen in children with indwelling central venous catheters (e.g. for parenteral nutrition or chemotherapy).

The child presents with fever, malaise and anorexia. Signs include clubbing, splinter haemorrhages in the nails and splenomegaly, and the pre-existing heart murmur may change in character. Microscopic haematuria may be found. The diagnosis is made on blood culture, and echocardiography, which shows vegetations on the heart valves. Intravenous antibiotics are required for 6 weeks.

Osteomyelitis

Osteomyelitis affects long bone metaphyses. Organisms are *Staphylococcus aureus*, *Haemophilus influenzae*, enterobacter species and *Streptococcus pyogenes*. Although the child may present with PUO, more usually the infected limb is obviously painful and held immobile. Swelling and redness eventually appear, and the adjacent joint may contain a sterile 'sympathetic' effusion. Repeated blood culture or direct aspiration of the bone abscess determines the causative organism. Radiographs are not helpful at presentation, as changes only become apparent after 10 days, but bone scans or MRI may be diagnostic. High-dose antibiotics are needed for up to 6 weeks, with surgical drainage if there is no immediate response. Inadequate treatment leads to bone necrosis, chronic discharge and limb deformity.

Serious recurrent infection and immunodeficiency

Most children experience recurrent trivial infections. These are commonly respiratory and peak on starting school or nursery. Despite parental concern they do not require investigation. However, recurrent serious infections or recurrent infections in an unusual site need to be thoroughly evaluated. There may be an anatomical cause (e.g. a fistula causing recurrent urinary tract infection, or splenectomy) or an inherited or acquired immunodeficiency.

Splenectomy and hyposplenism

Children who lack an effective spleen are at increased risk of sepsis, especially pneumococcal septicaemia. Hyposplenism may occur as a result of sickle cell disease (autoinfarction of the spleen) or after splenectomy for trauma, metabolic and haematological conditions (e.g. severe idiopathic thrombocytopenia purpura (ITP)). The risk of bacterial infection is especially high in children under 5 years old, and pneumococcal vaccination and prophylaxis with penicillin is recommended.

Congenital immunodeficiency

Most immunodeficiency disorders present in early childhood with recurrent infections and failure to thrive. In DiGeorge's syndrome there is cell-mediated immunodeficiency due to thymic aplasia, cardiac abnormality and hypoparathyroidism. Severe combined immunodeficiency (SCID) affects 1 in 100 000 and presents with opportunistic infection failure to thrive.

Acquired immunodeficiency

This is often due to side effects of chemotherapy or immunosuppressants following a transplant. It is important that those treating the child (e.g. primary care doctors) are aware of the risk of infections. Care should be taken to avoid contact with chickenpox, herpes simplex and other common infections.

HIV and AIDS

By far the commonest acquired immunodeficiency worldwide is HIV-1 infection leading to AIDS. 2.3 million children live with HIV, either infants born to infected mothers or adolescents who acquire infection sexually or by intravenous drug abuse. Young children usually present by the age of 3 years with failure to thrive, diarrhoea, recurrent oral candidiasis, hepatosplenomegaly, or severe bacterial infections.

Diagnosis is made by the detection of HIV antibody or viral load by PCR Techniques. Treatment uses combination highly active antiretroviral therapy (HAART), antibiotic prophylaxis with co-trimoxazole and appropriate viral vaccination. In developing countries affected children often die in infancy or early childhood, but in the UK, with early diagnosis and treatment, the prognosis is good, with most children achieving viral suppression (an undetectable viral load by HIV PCR tests).

Without intervention, vertical transmission is 20–30%. Viral load should be reduced in pregnancy with HAART and with use of zidovudine in labour and for 4 weeks after birth, delivery by caesarean section and avoidance of breast-feeding, it can be reduced to <2%. Breast-feeding doubles the risk of infection. Because maternal anti-HIV IgG antibody crosses the placenta, a standard HIV test is not reliable in the first 18 months of life, and a quantitative RNA/DNA must be used.

> **KEY POINTS**
>
> - A thorough history and repeat physical examinations are required. This may save the child from multiple investigations.
> - The characteristics of the fever may give a clue to diagnosis.
> - Samples for culture should be taken at the peak of the fever.
> - In severe, unusual or recurrent infections, consider immunodeficiency.

Causes of 'chestiness'

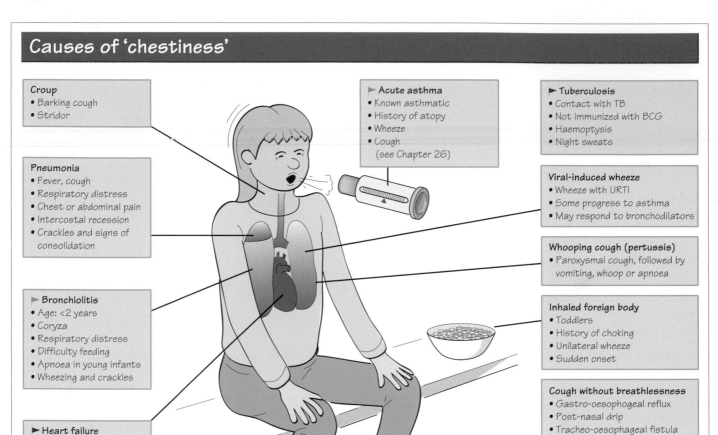

Croup
- Barking cough
- Stridor

Pneumonia
- Fever, cough
- Respiratory distress
- Chest or abdominal pain
- Intercostal recession
- Crackles and signs of consolidation

▶ **Bronchiolitis**
- Age: <2 years
- Coryza
- Respiratory distress
- Difficulty feeding
- Apnoea in young infants
- Wheezing and crackles

▶ **Heart failure**
- Left to right shunts, e.g. ASD, VSD

▶ **Acute asthma**
- Known asthmatic
- History of atopy
- Wheeze
- Cough (see Chapter 26)

▶ **Tuberculosis**
- Contact with TB
- Not immunized with BCG
- Haemoptysis
- Night sweats

Viral-induced wheeze
- Wheeze with URTI
- Some progress to asthma
- May respond to bronchodilators

Whooping cough (pertussis)
- Paroxysmal cough, followed by vomiting, whoop or apnoea

Inhaled foreign body
- Toddlers
- History of choking
- Unilateral wheeze
- Sudden onset

Cough without breathlessness
- Gastro-oesophageal reflux
- Post-nasal drip
- Tracheo-oesophageal fistula
- Passive smoking
- Cystic fibrosis

What you need from your evaluation

History

- Are there features of infection such as pyrexia or poor appetite?
- Is there a history of previous episodic breathlessness suggesting recurrent asthma?
- Is the child atopic—asthma, hayfever, eczema?
- Is there a relevant family history, e.g. asthma, cystic fibrosis, TB?
- Is there an underlying condition, such as congenital heart disease or prematurity, that increases the risk of severe bronchiolitis?

Examination

- Are there signs of respiratory distress—grunting, nasal flaring, intercostal recession, tachypnoea?
- Are there any additional noises—wheeze, stridor, cough?
- Are there signs of consolidation—reduced air entry, crackles, bronchial breathing, dullness on percussion and reduced expansion? (NB: signs are often not focal in young children)
- Are there signs of a chronic respiratory condition, e.g. finger clubbing, chest deformity?
- Is there evidence of congenital heart disease?
- Is the child cyanosed?
- Is the child pyrexial?
- Can the child talk in full sentences?
- Is the peak expiratory flow rate (PEFR) normal?

Investigations and their significance

• Chest radiograph	Focal consolidation suggests bacterial infection; diffuse suggests viral or atypical pneumonia. Hyperinflation in asthma and bronchiolitis. May be patchy collapse in bronchiolitis
• Full blood count	Neutrophilia in bacterial pneumonia Lymphocytosis in pertussis
• Sputum culture	To isolate causative organisms. Acid-fast bacilli may be seen in TB
• Nasopharyngeal aspirate	Viral immunofluorescence for RSV in bronchiolitis
• Per-nasal swab	To isolate Bordetella pertussis
• Viral titres	In atypical pneumonia, e.g. mycoplasma
• Blood cultures	In suspected bacterial pneumonia may isolate Streptococcus pneumoniae or Staphylococcus aureus
• Mantoux test	In suspected TB
• Bronchoscopy	Rigid bronchoscopy to remove foreign body or flexible to perform diagnostic bronchio-alveolar lavage

The 'chesty' child

Children commonly present with coryza, breathlessness, cough, wheeze or noisy breathing. This is often due to a viral URTI (see Chapter 21) or asthma (see Chapter 26).

Pneumonia

Pneumonia (lower respiratory tract infection), can be either bacterial or viral:
- Viral causes include respiratory syncytial virus (RSV), influenza, parainfluenza, adenovirus and Coxsackie virus.
- Bacterial causes are *Streptococcus pneumoniae*, *Haemophilus influenzae*, staphylococcus, *Mycoplasma pneumoniae* and, in the newborn, group B beta-haemolytic streptococcus.
- *Pseudomonas aeruginosa* and *Staphylococcus aureus* are more common in those with underlying respiratory disease, such as cystic fibrosis (see Chapter 27).
- Predisposing factors include a congenital anomaly of the bronchi, inhaled foreign body, immunosuppression, recurrent aspiration (e.g. with a tracheo-oesophageal fistula) or cystic fibrosis.

Pneumonia usually presents with a short history of fever, cough and respiratory distress, including tachypnoea and intercostal recession. Grunting is common in infants. Signs include dullness to percussion, bronchial breathing and crackles, reflecting the underlying consolidation. Clinical signs are often not reliable in infants and the diagnosis should always be confirmed by chest radiograph. This may show a lobar pneumonia or a more widespread bronchopneumonia.

Blood and sputum cultures may reveal the organism. Antibody titres may be useful in diagnosing mycoplasma pneumonia, which often has a more insidious onset and requires treatment with erythromycin. Penicillin is the first-line antibiotic for lobar pneumonia.

Complications of pneumonia include pleural effusion, septicaemia, bronchiectasis, empyema (infected pleural effusion) or lung abscess (may follow staphylococcal pneumonia).

Bronchiolitis

Bronchiolitis is an acute cause of respiratory distress and wheezing in infants, due to obstruction of the small airways. It is usually caused by RSV and occurs in epidemics in the winter months. RSV is highly infectious, and spreads rapidly in daycare nurseries. Adenovirus, influenza and parainfluenza virus can also cause bronchiolitis. Coryza is followed by cough, respiratory distress and wheeze. Some infants have difficulty feeding or may have apnoea. Examination reveals widespread wheeze and fine crackles and overexpansion of the chest. Chest radiograph will show hyperinflation and patchy collapse or consolidation. A nasopharyngeal aspirate (NPA) can identify RSV using immunofluoresence.

Most children do not require any specific treatment but indications for admission to hospital include poor feeding, apnoea, increasing respiratory distress or the need for oxygen. The illness usually lasts 7–10 days and most recover fully although there may be recurrent wheezing during infancy. A minority, particularly those with chronic lung disease or an underlying congenital heart defect, will require intensive care. There is no effective treatment other than oxygen, bronchodilators and supportive therapy. Bronchiolitis has a mortality of 1–2%. A monoclonal antibody (palivizumab) against RSV can be given prophylactically to high-risk infants throughout the winter months to provide passive immunity against infection.

Whooping cough

Bordetella pertussis pneumonia tends to occur in young infants or in those who are not fully vaccinated. Paradoxical coughing spasms during expiration are followed by a sharp intake of breath—the whoop. In infants it can cause apnoea. Diagnosis is mainly clinical, although a lymphocytosis ($>20 \times 10^9$/L) is suggestive. The organism may be cultured from a per-nasal swab. Treatment is supportive. The paroxysms of coughing can continue for months (the 100-day cough).

Croup (acute laryngotracheobronchitis)

This common condition affects children aged 6 months to 3 years and is due to a parainfluenza infection of all the upper airways. It is most common in winter and can be recurrent. Croup starts with coryzal symptoms, then proceeds to stridor (Chapter 24), wheeze and a barking cough. Children may have a hoarse voice. It is usually self-limiting but can occasionally be very severe, requiring intubation and ventilation. Signs of severe croup include increased work of breathing, cyanosis and restlessness. Milder cases can be managed by observation and maintaining good hydration. Nebulized budesonide and oral dexamethasone reduce the severity of symptoms and the need for hospital admission. Steam and humidity have not been proven to be beneficial but may provide some symptomatic relief.

Acute epiglottitis

This life-threatening infection is caused by *Haemophilus influenzae* and is now rare thanks to immunization with the Hib vaccine. It presents in children (2–4 years) with signs of sepsis and an inability to swallow or talk. Children often lean forwards to maintain a patent airway and may drool saliva. If epiglottitis is suspected, examination of the throat is contraindicated as it may precipitate complete airway obstruction. The child should be transferred immediately to an operating theatre for intubation by an experienced anaesthetist. At laryngoscopy a 'cherry red' swollen epiglottis confirms the diagnosis. Once the airway is protected, blood cultures can be taken and intrevenous antibiotics (cefotaxime) given.

KEY POINTS

- The majority of children with 'chestiness' have a self-limiting viral URTI and do not require antibiotics.
- If a child has recurrent episodes of pneumonia, an underlying cause should be sought.
- Bronchiolitis is very common in winter, especially among infants with chest or cardiac disease.
- Whooping cough is diagnosed by the characteristic paroxysmal cough and associated colour change.
- Croup causes a barking cough and stridor, usually following a coryzal illness.
- Epiglottitis is a life-threatening infection.

Chronic stridor   Acute stridor

Stridor is an inspiratory noise caused by narrowing of the upper airway outside of the thorax. It is a very common symptom in young children and infants, but in a minority of cases can represent life-threatening disorders such as inhaled foreign body or epiglottitis. It may be chronic, due to a congenital abnormality, or acute, usually due to infection or obstruction.

Laryngeal anomalies
- Vocal cord palsy: may be associated with brain lesions or trauma
- Papilloma: due to vertical transmission of wart virus. Causes progressive stridor

► Laryngomalacia (floppy larynx)
- Variable stridor from birth
- Loudest when crying, disappears when settled
- Caused by prolapse of the aryepiglottic folds into upper larynx
- Usually resolves within a few months
- A well, thriving baby with characteristic mild stridor does not need investigations
- If stridor is progressive, interfering with feeding or causing respiratory distress then microlaryngo-bronchoscopy is indicated

Upper airway obstruction
- Severe micrognathia (e.g. Pierre Robin syndrome)
- Pharyngeal cysts

Tracheal abnormalitiy
- Subglottic stenosis—following prolonged intubation
- Tracheomalacia—abnormality of cartilage ring which may lead to recurrent lobar collapse

Vascular ring
- Congenital abnormality of great vessels (e.g. double aortic arch)
- Worsens over time, may have feeding difficulties
- Barium swallow shows indentation
- High resolution CT scan is needed to plan corrective surgery

► Croup (see Chapter 23)
- Infection of larynx or trachea
- Usually viral
- Coryzal illness
- Barking cough

Tonsillar abscess (quinsy)

► Anaphylaxis (see Chapter 54)

► Epiglottitis (see Chapter 23)
- Sudden onset
- Septic
- Painful swallowing
- Drooling
- Muffled voice
- May have missed Hib vaccine

► Inhaled foreign body
- Toddlers
- Sudden onset
- History of choking
- Unilateral signs
- Requires bronchoscopy

What you need from your evaluation

History

- How long has the stridor been present? In a well baby stridor that comes and goes and has been present from birth is usually due to laryngomalacia (floppy larynx), which usually improves with time. Persistent fixed stridor may be due to a vascular ring or, more rarely, vocal cord palsy, or severe micrognathia (e.g. Pierre Robin sequence)
- Does the child look acutely ill? The most common cause of stridor is croup—it is often worse at night and associated with a barking cough and preceding coryzal symptoms. Always consider epiglottitis, which presents more quickly in a very ill child who cannot swallow or speak and is a life-threatening emergency
- In any child with sudden onset of stridor, ask about choking as an inhaled foreign body must always be considered
- Is there any history of allergy that would suggest anaphylaxis?

Examination

- Assess the severity by the work of breathing, the presence of intercostal recession and the degree of oxygenation (by colour or by saturation monitoring if available)
- Unilateral wheeze or chest hyperexpansion suggests an inhaled foreign body
- An urticarial rash and angioedema suggest anaphylaxis
- If the child is sitting forwards, unable to swallow and is acutely unwell, consider epiglottitis—in this instance do not try to examine the throat until the airway has been secured. Call for senior anaesthetic help before examining the child
- In chronic stridor assess the shape and size of the jaw. Listen for murmurs which may suggest congenital heart disease, where abnormal great vessels can compress the airways

Investigations and their significance

Investigations will be determined by the likely diagnosis as follows:
- Foreign body   Chest radiograph for unilateral hyperexpansion or radio-opaque objects
                    Rigid bronchoscopy to find and retrieve the object
- Croup   Usually none required
- Epiglottitis   Do not perform investigations until airway secured!
                    Blood culture and FBC
- Persistent stridor Microlaryngoscopy (if infant not thriving or stridor very severe) to assess larynx and vocal cords
                    Barium swallow (may show indentation of vascular ring)

Key points

- Stridor suggests upper airway obstruction
- Always consider an inhaled foreign body
- Acute epiglottitis is a life-threatening infection
- Croup responds to corticosteroid therapy

Causes of swellings in the neck

Mastoiditis
- Tender inflamed swelling behind ear
- Ear pushed out
- Complication of otitis media
- Medical emergency: can cause meningitis or sinus thrombosis
- Requires IV antibiotics and sometimes surgical mastoidectomy

Parotid gland: mumps
- Swelling overlies the angle of the jaw
- Ear displaced up and outward
- Unilateral or bilateral
- Fever and malaise
- Pain on swallowing sweet or sour liquids

Thyroid gland: thyroiditis
- Anterior midline swelling
- Smooth, diffusely enlarged, non-tender
- Insidious onset
- May be clinically hypothyroid, hyperthyroid or normal
- Thyroid function tests abnormal with thyroid autoantibody present

Lymph glands
▶ **Cervical adenitis**
- Tender swollen glands, usually along anterior cervical chain
- Unilateral or bilateral
- Acutely unwell
- Fever, sore throat
- High white cell count

▶ **Infectious mononucleosis** (see Chapter 21)
- Fever, sore throat
- Large purulent tonsils
- Generalized lymphadenopathy and splenomegaly
- Due to EBV
- Atypical lymphocytes on blood film

▶ **Lymphoma**
- Firm, non-tender nodes
- Immobile or matted
- Malaise, night sweats, persistent fever
- Hepatosplenomegaly
- Weight loss

Atypical mycobacterium
- Mycobacterium avium intracellulare infection
- Cervical lymphadenitis
- Diagnosis by culture or biopsy
- Treat with clarithromycin and ethambutol

What you need from your evaluation

History
- Ask about malaise and sore throat
- What is the duration of the illness?
- In the case of thyroid swelling, ask about symptoms of hypothyroidism (tiredness, constipation, underachievement at school) or hyperthyroidism (hyperactivity, increased appetite, palpitations, heat intolerance)

Physical examination
- **Identify the site of the swelling:**
  - Lymph nodes usually lie along the anterior cervical chain
  - Parotid glands overlie the angle of the jaw, with displacement of the ear up and out
  - The thyroid is midline anteriorly, and best palpated by standing behind the child
  - The mastoid is behind the ear and pushes the ear out
- **Palpate the gland.** Infected glands are mobile and tender. Malignant glands are fixed and matted
- Look for other sites of infection, e.g. tonsillitis, otitis media
- If the child is acutely unwell, look for signs of dehydration
- If cervical lymphadenopathy is present look for generalized lymphadenopathy and hepatosplenomegaly
- In the case of thyroid swelling, determine if the child is hypothyroid (poor growth, low pulse and BP, delayed tendon reflexes), hyperthyroid (tremor, sweating, fast pulse, high BP, eye signs) or euthyroid

Investigations and their significance

Cervical lymph nodes	FBC	High white cell count in bacterial infection; atypical lymphocytes in infectious mononucleosis
	EBV screen	Positive in infectious mononucleosis
	Throat culture	Group A haemolytic streptococcal infection needs antibiotics
Parotid glands	Serum or urine amylase	Elevated in mumps, but not usually required for diagnosis
Thyroid gland	T4 TSH	To assess if child is hypo-, hyper- or euthyroid
	Thyroid antibodies	Often positive in thyroiditis
Mastoid process	Tympanocentesis	To identify responsible organism and drain infection

Key points
- Identify the gland involved
- If the process is thought to be infective, assess how sick the child is, and the state of hydration
- If cervical lymphadenopathy is identified, look for generalized lymphadenopathy and hepatosplenomegaly
- If a goitre is found, assess whether the child is hypo-, hyper- or euthyroid
- If mastoiditis is found, admit the child as an emergency

Chronic asthma

Cough
- Recurrent dry cough
- Worse at night
- Worse with exercise

Wheeze
- Expiratory noise due to airway narrowing
- Often triggered by viral infections
- Responds to bronchodilators

Shortness of breath
- Exercise limitation
- Triggers can be exercise, cold, allergens, smoke

Uncontrolled asthma
- Poor growth
- Chronic chest deformity
- Time off school
- Frequent acute exacerbations

Pathology
- Environmental triggers cause bronchoconstriction, mucosal oedema and excess mucus production in a genetically predisposed child
- Airway narrowing causes wheeze and shortness of breath

Acute asthma

► Acute asthma attack
- Acutely short of breath
- Cough and wheeze
- Work of breathing increased
- Child often frightened
- May be triggered by viral illness, exposure to allergens, exercise or cold air

Assessing severity

Mild
- Breathless but not distressed
- Peak expiratory flow rate (PEFR) reduced but still >50% of normal

Severe
- Too breathless to talk or feed
- Respiratory rate >50 breaths/min, pulse >130 beats/min
- PEFR <50% of expected

Life-threatening
- PEFR <33% of expected
- 'Silent chest' or cyanosis
- Fatigue, drowsiness, confusion
- Hypotension

What you need from your evaluation

History

- Ask about the cough and wheeze. What triggers it and at what time of day does it occur?
- How many acute exacerbations have there been? How severe was the worst attack?
- How does the asthma affect the child's life? Does it limit activities; has school been missed?
- How often has the child had to use reliever treatment? How effective was it?
- Are there other atopic symptoms such as hay fever (allergic rhinitis) or eczema or a family history of atopy?

Investigations and their significance

- PEFR — Peak expiratory flow rate is best recorded in a peak flow diary to monitor change over time
- Chest radiograph — To exclude pneumothorax in severe asthma. Avoid excessive radiographs
- Allergy tests — Skin prick test mot usually helpful. Specific IgE to common inhaled allergens may identify allergens to be avoided

Examination

- In well-controlled asthmatics there may be no physical signs between acute exacerbations
- Listen for wheeze. Beware the 'silent chest' of severe asthma when there is almost no air moving
- Look for chronic chest deformity: barrel chest and Harrison's sulcus in severe uncontrolled asthma
- Measure PEFR using handheld peak flow meter
- Check height and weight and plot on centile chart. Poorly controlled asthma stunts growth, as will overuse of oral corticosteroids
- Check inhaler technique periodically

Management

- Aim to control symptoms, prevent exacerbations and achieve best possible pulmonary function
- **Medication:** 'preventers' (inhaled steroids or leukotriene receptor antagonists) and 'relievers' (bronchodilators)
- **Environmental control:** avoid passive smoking and reduce house dust mite exposure if possible
- **Self-monitoring of disease severity:** PEFR and symptom diary, management plan for each child
- **Education:** of the child, the family and the school on good control of asthma, inhaler technique and emergency treatment of an acute exacerbation

Asthma is the commonest chronic illness of childhood, occurring in up to 15% of children. The symptoms of cough, wheeze and dyspnoea are due to narrowing of the bronchi and bronchioles, mucosal inflammation and thick mucus. In a susceptible individual this process is initiated by environmental factors such as dust mite allergens, air pollution, cigarette smoke, cold air, viral infections, stress and exercise.

Presentation

Children with asthma usually present in infancy or early childhood. The diagnosis is clinical, based on recurrent cough or wheeze that responds to bronchodilator treatment. A history of atopy (eczema or hay fever) or a family history of asthma supports the diagnosis. In infancy it is often unclear whether recurrent wheeze is the first manifestation of asthma or merely airway obstruction due to viral respiratory tract infections. As the airways are narrow, mucosal oedema contributes more to obstruction than bronchoconstriction, and there may be poor response to bronchodilators.

In older children recurrent episodes of wheeze and cough, especially if triggered by exercise, viral infections or allergens, suggest a diagnosis of asthma. A good response to bronchodilators, either in symptom reduction or improvement in peak expiratory flow rate (PEFR), confirms the diagnosis. In asthma the chest radiograph may show hyperinflation (due to air trapping) and areas of collapse (due to mucous plugging). Skin prick testing is not usually helpful. Blood can be sent for specific IgE to common inhaled allergens and may identify allergens to be avoided.

Management of chronic asthma

The goal of good asthma management is to relieve the symptoms and allow normal activity, school attendance and growth. A step-wise approach is used—increasing the amount of treatment until control is obtained, then stepping back to the minimum required to maintain good control.

| Metered dose inhaler | Spacer device | Dry powder device |

Inhaler devices

Treatment is effective only if the drug is delivered in sufficient quantity to the small airways of the lungs. This is best achieved using an aerosolized drug delivery system, via a metered dose inhaler (MDI). A high degree of coordination is required to activate the MDI during inhalation, and this method is really only suitable for teenagers.

For children under 5 years, the MDI can be used in conjunction with a spacer device (e.g. Aerochamber). In infants these should be fitted with a mask to place over the child's mouth and nose.

Medical management of asthma in children*

	<5 years	5–12 years
Step 1. Mild intermittent asthma		
	Inhaled short-acting β_2 agonist prn	Inhaled short-acting β_2 agonist prn
Step 2. Regular preventive therapy		
	Add inhaled steroids	Add inhaled steroids
Step 3. Add-on therapy (<6 months proceed to step 4)		
	Add leukotriene receptor antagonist	1. Add inhaled long-acting β_2 agonist (LABA) 2. Consider leukotriene receptor antagonist or oral theophylline
Step 4. Persistent poor control		
	Refer to respiratory paediatrician	Increase dose of inhaled steroids
Step 5. Persistent poor control		
	Not used	Add oral low-dose daily steroids Refer to respiratory paediatrician

In children aged 5–12 the choice of device includes MDI spacer or Dry Powder Inhaler, depending on preference for convenience and effectiveness. Nebulisers can be used for delivering high doses quickly, although there is evidence that MDIs via a spacer are as effective. Nebulizers can be used in infants and for emergency treatment of acute exacerbations although there is evidence that MDIs via a spacer are as effective.

Treatment of severe exacerbation

Acute exacerbations should be treated promptly at home by using more reliever medication. If symptoms continue or worsen then aggressive treatment with high flow oxygen, regular β_2-agonists or ipratropium bromide via a nebulizer or spacer device (e.g. 10 puffs) and systemic corticosteroids is indicated. All children should have oxygen saturations measured and be admitted for close observation. If the oxygen saturation in air is <92% following treatment then the child should be admitted to hospital. In life-threatening asthma an infusion of steroids, salbutamol or aminophylline is used.

KEY POINTS

• Asthma is the commonest chronic childhood illness, occurring in 10–15% of all children.
• Bronchoconstriction, viscid mucous and mucosal oedema cause airway narrowing with wheeze, cough and dyspnoea.
• Treatment is increased and decreased step by step to gain symptom control and maintain a normal lifestyle.
• It is crucial to use an inhaler device suitable for the child's age.

Ear, nose and throat
- Nasal polyps
- Sinusitis

Recurrent chest infections
- Cough
- Purulent sputum
- Pneumonia
- Chronic pseudomonas infection
- Bronchiectasis
- Chest deformity
- Eventual respiratory failure

Finger clubbing
- Seen with chronic lung infection

Liver disease
- Obstructive jaundice in neonatal period (rare)
- Biliary stasis may require treatment with ursodeoxycholic acid
- Eventually liver cirrhosis may develop

Airway clearance
- Regular chest physiotherapy
- Inhaled bronchodilators
- Nebulized dornase alfa can help thin viscid secretions by breaking down DNA strands within the mucus

High salt losses in sweat
- Salty taste to skin
- Risk of salt-losing crisis during very hot weather

Poor growth
- Require 40% extra energy intake compared with normal child
- Poor weight gain
- Short stature
- Normal growth is achievable with pancreatic replacement, and aggressive treatment of chest infections
- Malabsorption

Gastrointestinal effects
- Pancreatic insufficiency
- Poor fat absorption
- Steatorrhoea (fatty stools)
- Distended abdomen
- Rectal prolapse
- Distal intestinal obstruction syndrome (DIOS) – can mimic acute appendicitis
- Need to take pancreatic enzymes with food and drinks which contain fat
- May develop diabetes
- Meconium ileus at birth (15%)

Male infertility
- Congenital absence of the vas deferens

History

- May be a family history of cystic fibrosis, although most new diagnoses do not have a family history
- Failure to thrive with ravenous appetite
- Cough and wheeze
- Recurrent chest infections
- Recurrent sinusitis
- Bulky, pale, offensive smelling stools, often difficult to flush away
- Fall in lung function and weight loss may indicate onset of CF-related diabetes

Examination

- Finger clubbing
- Evidence of malnutrition, poor weight gain and poor growth
- Delayed puberty
- Nasal polyps
- Chest deformity (e.g. chronic hyperexpansion)
- Crackles on auscultation
- Firm enlarged liver (rare) and splenomegally
- Subcutaneous vascular access devices may be present
- Gastrostomy tube may be present

Chest radiograph of a boy with cystic fibrosis
There is gross overinflation of the lungs with hilar enlargement and ring shadows caused by bronchial wall thickening and bronchiectatic change

Cystic fibrosis (CF) is the commonest recessive genetic disorder in white populations of European origin. It causes a molecular defect in a cellular membrane chloride channel which leads to the production of excessively thick mucus in many body systems. The sweat is considerably saltier than normal (>60 mmol/L). There is no cure, but effective treatment can greatly improve the quality and length of life.

Genetics

CF is caused by a gene defect in the CF transmembrane regulator (*CFTR*) gene on chromosome 7. Over 1000 different mutations have been identified but 75% are due to a mutation known as ΔF508. The inheritance is autosomal recessive (see Chapter 8). To be affected by CF, children must inherit an abnormal *CFTR* gene from each parent. These may be two copies of the same mutation (homozygous) or two different CF-causing mutations (compound heterozygous). Carriers are unaffected. Some mutations may result in an atypical presentation and progression of the disease.

The abnormal CFTR channel in the cell membrane leads to production of excessively viscid secretions in the body. This leads to obstruction of the small and large airways and recurrent infection. Abnormal sweat gland function leads to excessive sodium and chloride in sweat, which can be measured to confirm the diagnosis. There is usually pancreatic exocrine failure and in males absence of the vas deferens leading to infertility.

Presentation

Children with CF may be diagnosed by screening soon after birth, or antenatally in affected families. 1 in 10 present with meconium ileus (obstruction due to viscid meconium in the newborn bowel). Others will have failure to thrive and malabsorption from infancy or may present with recurrent chest infections. Atypical cases may present much later.

Common problems and their management
Chest infections

Thick viscid mucus causes obstruction and predisposes to lung infection. Children may develop chronic respiratory infection, especially when colonized with *Pseudomonas aeruginosa* or *Burkholderia cepacia*. Infection with these bacteria can lead to a rapid deterioration in lung function, and cross-infection to other people with CF must be avoided (e.g. by avoiding mixing individuals with CF in the same clinic). Treatment may involve regular bronchodilators, antibiotics (oral, nebulized or intravenously, which can be delivered at home via an indwelling central line). Steroid therapy may be needed to suppress lung inflammation. Nebulized DNAse enzymes can help break down mucus in the lung.

Preventive physiotherapy includes regular airway clearance by a variety of techniques including exercise, autogenic drainage, positive expiratory pressure, inhalation therapy and postural awareness. Prophylactic immunization against influenza and pneumococcus is recommended.

Malabsorption

Pancreatic failure means that fatty food cannot be broken down easily and causes steatorrhoea. This can lead to malnutrition and deficiency of fat-soluble vitamins (A, D, E, K). Taking pancreatic enzyme capsules with food can help with fat absorption and should be started even in babies. High-calorie diets may be required as children with CF have high metabolic demands. Fat-soluble vitamin supplements and advice from a specialist dietician are recommended.

Diabetes melitus

25% will develop impaired glucose tolerance. Optimization of blood glucose is associated with an improvement in lung function.

Salt loss

Salt supplementation may be required to replace sweat losses. This must be carefully monitored, especially in infancy where excessive salt intake can be dangerous.

Liver disease

Sluggish bile flow may cause biliary disease and rarely cirrhosis. Ursodeoxycholic acid can help. Children with CF may develop 'pseudo-obstruction' of the bowel which can easily be mistaken for appendicitis but usually responds to adjustment of pancreatic enzyme replacement or osmotic laxatives and does not require surgery.

Subfertility

Most men with cystic fibrosis have absence of the vas deferens leading to infertility. Assisted conception techniques can help. Women may be subfertile but most women with CF can achieve conception. Carrier testing of partners should be considered. Antenatal diagnosis of CF is possible via chorionic villus biopsy or amniocentesis.

Diagnosis

• **Newborns:** may be diagnosed by newborn bloodspot screening (see Chapter 8). Immunoreactive trypsin levels are elevated in affected babies. There is a better prognosis if CF can be diagnosed before it causes symptoms.
• **Gene testing:** Children presenting with a typical history or detected by screening should be diagnosed by mutation analysis of the *CFTR* gene. A panel of mutations are assessed but these routinely include only 30 of over 1000 mutations. Non-white families may have unusual variants which can be missed.
• **Sweat test:** This is the diagnostic test for CF and requires measuring sodium and chloride concentration in sweat, collected by passing a small electric current across the skin.

Prognosis

There is presently no cure for CF. The prognosis has improved enormously in the last 25 years with aggressive nutritional and respiratory support, and more than half of affected children live beyond the age of 38 years. Lung function tests (e.g. FEV_1) are the best measure of disease progression. Lung or heart–lung transplantation is offered to those with end-stage respiratory disease. Some individuals have survived 15 years following transplantation.

Causes of acute abdominal pain

▶Mesenteric adenitis
- Recent viral infection
- No peritonism
- Pain can mimic appendicitis

▶Intussusception
- Intermittent screaming/colic
- Shock/pallor
- 'Redcurrant jelly' stool
- Usually 3–24 months old

Inflammatory bowel disease
- Blood/mucus in stools
- Family history of diarrhoea
- Weight loss and poor growth

▶Diabetes
- Diabetic ketoacidosis

Acute appendicitis
- Anorexia
- Central pain localizing to right iliac fossa
- Peritonism in right iliac fossa
- Tachycardia

Lower lobe pneumonia
- Signs of pneumonia
- Referred abdominal pain

Peptic ulcer
- Pain at night
- Relief with milk
- Helicobacter pylori

Henoch–Schönlein purpura
- Purpuric rash on legs
- Joint pain

Urinary tract infection
- Dysuria, frequency
- Bedwetting
- Back pain
- Vomiting
- Evidence of infection on urinalysis or microscopy

Constipation
- Hard or infrequent stools
- Mass in left iliac fossa
- Faecal loading on radiograph

▶Intestinal obstruction
- Bile-stained vomiting
- Abdominal distension
- Consider a volvulus

Renal calculi
- Hydronephrosis

▶Gastroenteritis
- Vomiting and diarrhoea

What you need from your evaluation

History

- Pain in young children may present with intermittent unexplained screaming. Pallor and screaming are suggestive of intussusception. Older children may point to the site of pain. Pain migrating from the periumbilical area to the right iliac fossa suggests appendicitis. Sometimes children experience referred abdominal pain with lower lobe pneumonia
- Blood in the stool is a serious sign and may indicate intussusception, but also occurs in inflammatory bowel disease, Henoch–Schönlein purpura and some types of gastroenteritis
- It is important to ask about associated features such as vomiting, diarrhoea, recent viral infection, joint or urinary symptoms
- Loss of appetite (anorexia) is a particular feature of appendicitis
- Vomiting bile is highly suggestive of small bowel obstruction

Examination

- Examination should include an assessment of how ill the child looks and measurement of pulse, capillary refill time and temperature
- The abdomen should be palpated very gently at first, while watching the child's face for signs of pain
- Signs of peritonism are a reluctance to move, rebound tenderness, guarding and rigidity
- In mesenteric adenitis there is often palpable lymphadenopathy elsewhere

Investigations and their significance

- Full blood count — Leucocytosis found in acute appendicitis and urinary tract infection

- Urine dipstix test — Nitrite test positive in urinary tract infection. Haematuria sometimes seen with HSP

- Urine microscopy and culture — Pyuria and presence of organisms indicate infection

- Abdominal radiograph — Dilated bowel loops: intestinal obstruction. Abnormal gas pattern: intussusception. Faecal loading: constipation

- Abdominal ultrasound scan — To exclude renal tract abnormality and can be very useful in diagnosis of intussusception

- Barium enema/ air enema — For diagnosis and treatment of intussusception

- CRP/ESR — May be elevated in infection and in inflammatory bowel disease

Acute abdominal pain is very common. It is important to quickly assess whether surgical intervention is required, as some important surgical conditions present as an acute abdomen.

Acute appendicitis

This occurs in 3–4 per 1000 children and can present at any age, especially beyond 5 years of age, and is difficult to diagnose in very young children. In older children the pain is typically periumbilical and moves over a few hours to the right iliac fossa. There is loss of appetite and a reluctance to move. The most reliable signs are pain on movement and tenderness in the right iliac fossa due to peritonitis. There is often constipation, occasionally diarrhoea and vomiting and usually a low-grade fever. Investigations may show leucocytosis and neutrophilia. Urine should be checked to exclude infection. Abdominal radiograph is not helpful but CT scan or ultrasound is performed if the diagnosis is in doubt or an appendix abscess is suspected.

The differential diagnosis of iliac fossa pain includes:
- Mesenteric adenitis
- Gastroenteritis
- Constipation
- Urinary tract infection
- Henoch–Schönlein purpura (HSP)
- Inflammatory bowel disease
- Ovarian pain
- Ectopic pregancy
- Pyelonephritis.

Treatment is appendicectomy. This can be performed laparoscopically and has an excellent prognosis. Perforation is commoner in children. If peritonitis has occurred there may be severe illness and adhesions may later cause bowel obstruction.

Intussusception

Intussusception

Intussusception is the telescoping of one part of bowel into another; usually the ileum into the caecum (75%). It is commonest between 3 and 24 months; only 10% occur in children >3 years of age. Enlarged lymphatics may form the leading edge of the intussusception and this often follows a viral infection (adenovirus or rotavirus). Very rarely it is due to a pathological lesion such as a polyp or lymphoma or as a complication of HSP.

The child presents with episodic screaming and pallor and between episodes may appear well. There may be shock or dehydration. Passage of blood and mucus in the stool ('redcurrant jelly' stool) occurs in 75%, but is a late sign. A sausage-shaped mass may be palpable.

Abdominal radiograph may show the rounded edge of the intussusception against the gas-filled lumen of the distal bowel, with signs of proximal bowel obstruction. Ultrasound can confirm the presence of bowel within bowel—the 'doughnut sign'. The intussusception can often be reduced by an air or barium enema. If this fails or there is evidence of peritonitis then a laparotomy is required.

Children still die of intussusception because it can present non-specifically and the diagnosis is not always considered.

Other surgical causes of acute abdominal pain

Ovarian cysts

Ovarian cysts can be present even in prepubertal children and are present in 20% of teenage girls. They are usually asymptomatic but can cause severe pain with torsion, rupture or bleeding into the cyst. Mittleschmerz occurs in mid menstrual cycle due to rupture of a follicular cyst.

Volvulus

This is torsion of a malrotated intestine and presents with severe abdominal pain and bilious vomiting. Urgent surgery is required to untwist the volvulus and treat the underlying malrotation. If missed, the bowel may infarct.

Renal, ureteric and biliary stones

Stones cause severe colicky pain but are relatively rare in childhood, unless there is an underlying metabolic or haemolytic disorder.

Non-surgical causes of acute abdominal pain

- Colicky abdominal pain is a very common feature of gastroenteritis (Chapter 30) and may precede vomiting and diarrhoea by some hours.
- In sexually active girls, pelvic inflammatory disease and ectopic pregnancy should be considered. A pregnancy test and ultrasound may be indicated.
- Urinary tract infection, (pyelonephritis) can cause abdominal pain more than dysuria (see Chapter 34).
- Diabetic ketoacidosis may characteristically cause abdominal pain and vomiting (Chapter 18).
- Lower lobe pneumonia may cause pain referred to the abdomen.
- HSP causes abdominal pain due to widespread vasculitis (Chapter 53) and these children are at risk of intussusception.

Abdominal pain is a common symptom of anxiety and school refusal (Chapter 12).

Mesenteric adenitis

Mesenteric adenitis is caused by inflammation of intra-abdominal lymph nodes following an upper respiratory tract infection or gastroenteritis. The enlarged nodes cause acute pain which can mimic appendicitis, but there is no peritonism or guarding and there may be evidence of infection in the throat or chest. It is a diagnosis of exclusion and treatment is with simple analgesia.

Causes of vomiting

Newborn and infants

Overfeeding
• Feeding >200 mL/kg per day

▶ **Gastro-oesophageal reflux**
• Due to lax gastro-oesophageal sphincter: positional vomiting
• May lead to oesophagitis or aspiration pneumonia
• May cause apnoea and failure to thrive

▶ **Pyloric stenosis**
• 4–6 weeks old
• Projectile vomiting after feed
• Hungry after vomiting
• Constipated
• Palpable pyloric mass

Whooping cough
• Paroxysmal cough

▶ **Small bowel obstruction**
(congenital atresia or malrotation)
• Bile-stained vomiting
• Presents soon after birth
• May have abdominal distension

Constipation

Systemic infection
• Meningitis
• UTI (pyelonephritis)

Older children and adolescents

▶ **Gastroenteritis**
• Usually with diarrhoea
• History of contact with infection
• Check for dehydration
• Usually self-limiting

Migraine
• Characteristic headache

▶ **Raised intracranial pressure**
• Effortless vomiting
• Usually neurological signs
• Papilloedema

Bulimia: self-induced vomiting as part of an eating disorder

Toxic ingestion or medications

Pregnancy

What you need from your evaluation

History

• In infants it is important to differentiate posseting from serious vomiting. With significant vomiting the child will look ill and be failing to gain weight or may even be losing weight
• Take a thorough feeding history, as overfeeding is not uncommon in a thriving baby who seems hungry but vomits the excess milk after a feed
• Always ask about projectile vomiting (pyloric stenosis) and bile-stained vomiting. The latter suggests intestinal obstruction and must be investigated urgently
• The presence of diarrhoea suggests gastroenteritis
• Fever suggests infection, and it is important to look for infection outside the gastrointestinal system; UTI, otitis media and meningitis may all present with vomiting. Vomiting with infection tends not to be projectile
• Paroxysms of coughing followed by turning red or blue and vomiting suggests whooping cough
• Gastro-oesophageal reflux should be suspected in infants and children with disability such as Down's syndrome or cerebral palsy

Examination

• Check for dehydration, especially with gastroenteritis
• Feel for a palpable pyloric mass in any young infant
• Check for abdominal distension, which suggests intestinal obstruction
• Check for papilloedema and hypertension in cases of unexplained vomiting to exclude raised ICP as a cause
• Look for signs of meningitis

Investigations and their significance

Investigations are required only in particular cases:
• Plasma urea and electrolytes — To assess electrolyte imbalance in dehydration and in pyloric stenosis
• Plasma chloride, pH and bicarbonate — To assess degree of metabolic alkalosis in pyloric stenosis
• pH monitoring and barium swallow — May show significant gastro-oesophageal reflux
• Upper gastrointestinal contrast study — Mandatory in bile-stained vomiting in newborn to exclude malrotation

Regurgitating a small amount of milk, known as posseting, is normal in babies. Vomiting refers to more complete emptying of the stomach. Vomiting is one of the commonest symptoms in childhood, and is often due to gastroenteritis. It may be associated with more serious infections such as pyelonephritis, or may be the presenting symptom of life-threatening conditions such as meningitis or pyloric stenosis. In newborn infants bile-stained vomiting suggests a congenital intestinal obstruction, such as duodenal or ileal atresia or volvulus of a malrotated intestine. These need urgent investigation with an upper gastrointestinal (GI) contrast study.

Gastro-oesophageal reflux

Gastro-oesophageal reflux (GOR) is a common symptom in babies and in some older children with cerebral palsy or Down's syndrome. It is especially common in the preterm. It is due to weakness of the functional gastro-oesophageal sphincter which normally prevents stomach contents refluxing into the oesophagus. GOR may present with trivial posseting or significant oesophagitis, apnoea or even aspiration. Vomiting is worse after feeds and on lying down, and may occasionally cause failure to thrive. Abnormal posturing may occur with severe acid reflux—this is known as Sandifer's syndrome and can be mistaken for seizures.

GOR is usually diagnosed clinically on the basis of a typical history. Investigations should only be performed if the reflux is significant. These include a barium swallow and monitoring the oesophageal pH for 24 hours using a pH probe. The presence of acid in the oesophagus usually reflects reflux of stomach acid and the percentage of time that this occurs can be calculated over 24 hours. Endoscopy is used to confirm oesophagitis. Simple reflux can be managed by nursing the infant in a more upright position and by thickening the feeds with thickening agents (carob flour, or rice-flour thickeners). Formula milk is now available which thickens on contact with stomach acid, which can be helpful. Breast-fed infants may be helped by taking Gaviscon before a feed. Winding the baby well after feeds is important. In very severe reflux, drugs that affect gastric emptying and gut motility can be used and a small number of children with recurrent aspiration require surgical fundoplication. Most gastro-oesophageal reflux resolves over time as the infant sits upright more and is weaned on to a more solid diet.

Pyloric stenosis

Pyloric stenosis is caused by hypertrophy of the pylorus muscle. It usually develops in the first 2–8 weeks of life and is said to be most common in first-born male infants. It occurs in 1 in 300 to 1 in 500 newborn infants, and is the commonest indication for surgery in infancy. The vomiting increases in intensity and is characteristically projectile, occurring immediately after a feed. The vomitus is not bile-stained and the infant is usually hungry. There may be a history of constipation. Examination shows weight loss and dehydration and the infant is irritable due to hunger. Careful palpation after a test feed with the left hand, from the left side of the body reveals a hard mobile mass to the right of the epigastric area. Prominent peristaltic waves may be visible over the stomach. If there is doubt ultrasound examination shows a thickened and elongated pyloric muscle. Blood tests typically show a low plasma chloride, potassium and sodium, and a metabolic alkalosis second-ary to protracted vomiting of stomach acid. The infant should be fully rehydrated with careful correction of the electrolyte imbalance before definitive surgery is performed. Rehydration may take at least 24 hours. Surgery involves splitting the pylorus muscle without cutting through the mucosa (Ramstedt's pyloromyotomy). Laparoscopic pyloromyotomy is sometimes performed. Oral feeds can usually be commenced soon after surgery.

Vomiting due to gastroenteritis

Gastroenteritis (discussed in Chapter 30) is by far the commonest cause of vomiting in childhood, and is usually part of a gastrointestinal illness with diarrhoea. Viral gastroenteritis may sometimes cause vomiting without associated diarrhoea. This is typical of norovirus infection, which causes fever, myalgia, abdominal cramps and vomiting for 24–48 hours. Acute food poisoning or food allergy may also cause sudden vomiting.

Bowel obstruction

Bile-stained vomiting in the first days of life should always be investigated urgently. It may be due to congenital duodenal or ileal atresia or malrotation of the small bowel. Duodenal atresia is more common in Down's syndrome. Other causes of bowel obstruction include Hirshprung's disease (colonic aganglionosis) and meconium ileus (in cystic fibrosis). In older infants intussusception should be suspected (see Chapter 28). All newborn infants with bile-stained vomiting should have a nasogastric tube passed to aspirate the stomach and feeds should be stopped pending investigation with an upper GI contrast study. In congenital malrotation the small bowel is rotated on its mesentery and a Doppler ultrasound scan may show malalignment of the mesenteric vessels. Once the cause of the obstruction has been identified and the child has been rehydrated, definitive surgery can take place. In older children bowel obstruction may be secondary to adhesions from previous abdominal surgery (e.g. appendicectomy).

Sepsis presenting with vomiting

In young infants the signs of sepsis may be very non-specific. In an unwell infant with vomiting, urinary tract infection or early meningitis should always be considered.

Vomiting due to raised intracranial pressure

If an older child has a history of regular vomiting for more than a few days then raised intracranial pressure (e.g. due to a brain tumour) must be excluded by careful neurological examination including examination of the optic discs. Early morning vomiting is said to be typical of raised intracranial pressure.

> ### KEY POINTS
>
> - Vomiting is often due to infection or gastroenteritis.
> - Pyloric stenosis presents at 2–8 weeks with projectile vomiting.
> - Gastro-oesophageal reflux is common and usually responds to simply thickening the feeds.
> - Bile-stained vomiting in an infant is a serious symptom which always requires investigation.

Causes of dehydration

Excessive fluid loss

Excessive sweating
- High fever
- Hot climate
- Cystic fibrosis

Vomiting
- Pyloric stenosis
- Viral infections
- Gastroenteritis

▶ Acute diarrhoea
- Viral gastroenteritis
- Bacterial gastroenteritis
  shigella
  E. coli
  salmonella
  campylobacter
- Antibiotic-induced
- Food poisoning (toxins)
- Any acute infection

Fluid loss
- Burns
- Post surgery

Polyuria
- Diabetes mellitus, especially diabetic ketoacidosis

Inadequate intake

Inability to drink
- Herpes stomatitis
- Acute tonsillitis

▶ Inadequate access to water

What you need from your evaluation

History
- Has there been diarrhoea and/or vomiting?
- Is the vomiting projectile (pyloric stenosis)?
- How many loose stools have there been?
- Is the child passing less urine than normal? Ask when was the last wet nappy?
- How often and for how long has the child been vomiting?
- Does the child have cystic fibrosis or diabetes?

Investigations and their significance

(Investigations are required only in moderate to severe diarrhoea or if the child is very ill)

- U&E — For electrolyte imbalance and renal function
- Blood gas — Metabolic acidosis or alkalosis
- Urinalysis — For osmolality or specific gravity
- Blood sugar — To exclude diabetic ketoacidosis
- Stool culture — In gastroenteritis and food poisoning

Examination
- Weigh the child and compare with previous weight (if known) to assess dehydration
- In young infants feel for a pyloric mass during a test feed (pyloric stenosis)
- Assess the degree of dehydration (mild, moderate or severe) as follows:

	Mild	Moderate	Severe
Mouth and lips	Dry	Dry	Dry
Urine output	Normal	Reduced	None for 12 h
Mental state	Normal	Lethargic	Irritable or coma
Pulse rate	Normal	Tachycardia	Tachycardia
Blood pressure	Normal	Normal	Low
Capillary refill time	Normal	Delayed	Very delayed
Fontanelle	Normal	Sunken	Very sunken
Skin and eye turgor	Normal	Reduced	Very reduced
Dehydration (%)	<5	5–10	>10 (shock)

Treatment
- Use oral rehydration therapy where possible
- Treat shock with boluses of IV fluids
- Rehydrate slowly to replace fluid loss over at least 24 h
- Correct any electrolyte imbalance

Dehydration

Water accounts for up to 80% of an infant's weight. Loss of more than 5% of this water represents significant dehydration. Fluid may be depleted in the intracellular or extracellular compartments. If significant fluid is lost acutely from the intravascular part of the extracellular space, then shock may ensue. Normal body fluid is a balance between intake (drinking) and output (urine output, stool volume, sweat and insensible losses such as expiration). If intake does not keep up with losses, then the child becomes dehydrated. The commonest cause of dehydration in children is diarrhoea and vomiting due to gastroenteritis.

Acute diarrhoea

Episodes of acute diarrhoea are common in children, and are usually due to infection, although not always gastrointestinal (GI) infection. Dehydration due to gastroenteritis is sadly still a major cause of mortality in children in developing countries. Gastroenteritis is usually viral, and rotavirus is the main agent causing winter epidemics. Diarrhoea follows 1–2 days after low-grade fever, vomiting and anorexia. There may be acute abdominal pain and malaise. The diarrhoea resolves within a week and the management is adequate rehydration (see below). Bacterial gastroenteritis has a similar presentation and the common pathogens are *Escherichia coli,* shigella, salmonella and campylobacter. Meningism and febrile convulsions can occur with shigella, whilst bloody diarrhoea occurs in shigella and campylobacter infection.

Any infection or febrile illness can cause diarrhoea, especially in infants. This includes viral URTIs, chest infections, otitis media and UTI. Use of antibiotics may cause diarrhoea due to a disturbance of the normal enteric flora. Recurrence of diarrhoea on refeeding is most likely to be due to lactase deficiency and may require a lactose-free diet for a number of weeks.

Antibiotics should not be prescribed for uncomplicated gastroenteritis. Antiemetics and antimotility agents are not generally recommended. If there is evidence of septicaemia the child should be admitted for intravenous antibiotics. There is some evidence that the use of probiotics (e.g. lactobacillus species) may reduce the duration of diarrhoea. Breast-feeding should be continued whenever possible.

Management of dehydration

Try to determine the cause of the diarrhoea and the degree of dehydration. Ask about the duration of diarrhoea, whether there has been vomiting and when the child last passed urine.

The degree of dehydration can be assessed by the pulse, blood pressure, mucous membranes, urine output, skin turgor and by feeling the fontanelle (see box opposite).

In mild dehydration the only physical sign may be a dry mouth. 'Red flag' warning signs that may indicate likely progression to shock include sunken eyes, altered responsiveness, tachycardia, tachypnoea and reduced skin turgor (pinch test).

The child should be weighed, the difference between the weight at presentation and a recent weight can be used to estimate the volume of body water that has been lost (1 kg = 1 L). If the child is significantly dehydrated, blood should be taken for urea, electrolytes and bicarbonate and interpreted as in the table:

Finding	Interpretation
Metabolic acidosis	Bicarbonate loss in diarrhoea or shock with lactic acidosis
Metabolic alkalosis	Loss of H^+ ions from persistent vomiting in pyloric stenosis.
Hyponatraemia	Dehydration where diarrhoea contains high concentration of sodium ions. When $Na^+ < 130\,mmol/L$ the child is often lethargic and the skin feels dry and can be pinched into creases
Hypernatraemia	Dehydration where there is greater loss of water than sodium ions or excessive salt intake or excessively concentrated formula feeds. When $Na^+ > 150\,mmol/L$ the child is very thirsty and the skin may feel doughy.

Calculating the replacement and maintenance fluid requirements for intravenous rehydration

An infant weighing 7.5 kg is thought, on the basis of clinical examination, to be 10% dehydrated.

(A) If we assume the child is all water then 7.5 kg water = 7500 mL. 10% of this is 750 mL (fluid deficit).

(B) Maintenance fluids = 100 mL/kg per day for the first 10 kg of body weight, 50 mL/kg for next 10 kg and 20 mL/kg thereafter.

$$= 100 \times 7.5\ kg = 750\ mL$$

Deficit + maintenance = A + B, i.e. this child needs 750 + 750 = 1500 mL fluids over the first 24 hours to rehydrate and then maintain normal hydration.

Note: maintenance fluids covers essential urine output and insensible losses. If there are significant ongoing losses (e.g. diarrhoea) this volume may need to be increased further. The best initial maintenance fluid is 0.9%saline with 5% dextrose. The electrolyte content can be adjusted once serum electrolytes are known.

• **Mild dehydration (<5%):** may be treated at home using oral rehydration therapy, as long as the child is not vomiting excessively. The child should be encouraged to drink a rehydration solution which contains glucose and salt in the correct concentration to aid water absorption and restore electrolyte balance. Breast-feeding should be continued, but if the infant is formula fed, milk can be reintroduced once the diarrhoea has settled.

• **Moderate and severe dehydration:** It is just as effective, and usually safer, to rehydrate using oral rehydration solution (initially 50 mL/kg) orally or via a nasogastric tube. The volume of fluid necessary to correct the deficit of water and to provide maintenance fluids and cover ongoing losses is given over 24 hours (see box). If there is persistent vomiting then intravenous rehydration may be required. If shock is present give a 20 mL/kg bolus of intravenous 0.9% saline. Too-rapid intravenous rehydration can lead to dangerous fluid shifts and hyponatraemia.

Causes of chronic or recurrent diarrhoea

Frequent stools are often normal in early childhood. Babies have one to seven loose stools per day, which become formed and adult-like in odour and colour after 12 months of age. If the child is thriving and there are no other symptoms or signs, investigations are rarely necessary. Pathological diarrhoeal illnesses can broadly be divided into malabsorption, inflammation and infections.

NON-PATHOLOGICAL

► **Toddler diarrhoea**
• Thriving toddler
• Loose stools containing undigested food
• May have a large fluid intake
• Fast gut transit time

► **Non-specific diarrhoea**
• Loose watery stools
• Thriving child, may follow on from acute gastroenteritis

MALABSORPTION

Cystic fibrosis (see Chapter 27)
• Starts in infancy
• Failure to thrive with chest infections
• Fatty stools
• Diagnosis by sweat test

► **Coeliac disease**
• Failure to thrive with irritability
• Muscle wasting, abdominal distension
• Often presents after introduction of wheat into diet
• Fatty stools
• Diagnosis by jejunal biopsy

Secondary lactose intolerance
• Baby or toddler
• Follows acute gastroenteritis
• Watery stools with low pH and reducing substances

INFECTION

Parasites: *Giardia lamblia*
• Weight loss and abdominal pain
• Watery stools
• Common in nurseries

OTHER

Overflow diarrhoea in constipation
• Soiling rather than diarrhoea
• Constipated stool palpable abdominally or rectally

INFLAMMATION (rare)

► **Crohn's disease**
• Late childhood and adolescence
• Weight loss and abdominal pain
• Anorexia and fatigue
• Exacerbations and remissions

Cow's milk protein intolerance
• Occurs in babies
• Watery stools, may be bloody
• May have urticaria, stridor or bronchospasm, eczema

► **Ulcerative colitis**
• Late childhood and adolescence
• Bloody stools and abdominal pain
• Exacerbations and remissions

What you need from your evaluation

History

• **Bowel pattern.** Get an idea of the volume, appearance and consistency of the stools. Is there blood or mucus? A diary is helpful in assessing severity and pattern of symptoms. NB Odour and 'flushability' are usually not helpful
• **Precipitating factors.** Lactose intolerance is precipitated by acute diarrhoea. Are certain foods troublesome? Are others in the family or nursery affected?
• **Associated symptoms.** Weight loss or abdominal pain are particularly significant
• **Review of symptoms.** Non GI diseases may cause diarrhoea and failure to thrive

Investigations

• These are rarely necessary if a child is thriving and there are no accompanying symptoms or signs detailed investigations are listed opposite.

Physical examination

• **Growth.** Obtain height, weight, head circumference and compare with earlier measurements. Weight is useful as a baseline if symptoms persist. If growth is impaired consider chronic disease as a cause
• **Other features.** Hydration, pallor, abdominal distension, tenderness and finger clubbing are particularly relevant
• **General examination.** Does the child look ill? Look for non GI diseases which might cause diarrhoea
• **Anorectal examination.** Not routinely indicated

Blood

• Full blood count	Anaemia indicates blood loss, malabsorption, poor diet or inflammation (as in Crohn's disease) Eosinophilia suggests parasites or atopy
• Plasma viscosity/ ESR	High in inflammatory bowel disease
• Coeliac antibodies	A test for coeliac disease (requires confirmation by jejunal biopsy)

Other

• Urine culture	Urinary tract infection
• Sweat test	Cystic fibrosis
• Breath hydrogen test	High H_2 in carbohydrate maldigestion
• Jejunal biopsy	Subtotal villous atrophy with crypt hyperplasia in coeliac disease
• Barium follow through	Characteristic signs in small bowel Crohn's disease
• Endoscopy	Characteristic lesions on histology in inflammatory bowel disease

Stool

• Occult blood	Positive in colitis e.g. inflammatory bowel disease
• Ova and parasites (3 samples required)	Parasitic infection
• Reducing substances and low pH	Present in sugar intolerance (usually lactose)
• Fecal elastase	Low in pancreatic insufficiency
• Microscopy for fat globules	Globules seen in fat malabsorption/maldigestion (usually pancreatic insufficiency)
• Fecal calprotectin	Present in inflammatory bowel disease

Toddler diarrhoea

Toddlers often experience non-specific diarrhoea, probably due to a rapid gastrocolic reflex. Features are drinking excessive fluids, particularly fruit juices, and food particles in the stool. The diagnosis should only be made if the child is thriving. Reassurance is all that is required.

Lactose intolerance

Lactose intolerance is common in babies and young children following gastroenteritis. The superficial mucosal cells containing lactase are stripped off, causing high levels of lactose in the bowel, which prolongs the diarrhoea. Congenital lactose intolerance is rare. Lactose intolerance should be suspected if diarrhoea persists for weeks after a gastroenteritis illness. It is rarely necessary to perform lactose challenge or hydrogen breath tests. In bottle-fed babies an empirical change of formula to soy milk (which contains non-lactose sugar) can be tried. The baby should revert to cow's milk once symptoms resolve. Breast-fed babies should continue breastfeeding.

Coeliac disease

Coeliac disease results from intolerance to gluten, a substance found in wheat, rye and barley. Children usually present before 2 years of age with failure to thrive, irritability, anorexia, vomiting and diarrhoea. Signs include abdominal distension, wasted buttocks, irritability and pallor. The stools are pale and foul-smelling.

Investigations show iron deficiency anaemia and steatorrhoea. Coeliac antibodies (IgA anti-tissue transglutaminase or anti-endomysial antibodies) are present in blood, but a definitive diagnosis is made by finding subtotal villous atrophy on jejunal biopsy. Treatment is a gluten-free diet, eliminating all wheat and rye products. Improved mood, resolution of diarrhoea and good growth occur promptly. The diet is quite restrictive and must be continued indefinitely. Rechallenge with gluten after 2 years (to allow for full regeneration of the villi) and repeat biopsy are recommended. Coeliac disease is common—about 1 in 100 adults. It is associated with diabetes and Down's syndrome.

Inflammatory bowel disease

Inflammatory bowel disease (IBD) is a cause of chronic diarrhoea in late childhood and adolescence. Both Crohn's disease and ulcerative colitis are characterized by unpredictable exacerbations and remissions.

• **Crohn's disease** presents with recurrent abdominal pain, anorexia, growth failure, fever, diarrhoea, anaemia, oral and perianal ulcers and arthritis. Diagnosis is by endoscopic biopsy. Remission can be induced by an elemental diet, immunomodulator drugs, anti-TNF-alpha agents (infliximab) or steroids. Surgical resection may be indicated for localized disease.

• **Ulcerative colitis** presents with bloody diarrhoea and abdominal pain. Weight loss, arthritis and liver disturbance may also occur. Treatment is with oral or rectal mesalazine or steroid enemas. Immunosuppressive therapy, infliximab or even colectomy may be required in severe cases.

Parasites

Giardia lamblia can cause outbreaks of diarrhoea in daycare nurseries or may follow travel abroad. The child may be asymptomatic or have diarrhoea, weight loss and abdominal pain. Diagnosis is made on microscopic examination of the stool. Three separate specimens are required as excretion of the cysts can be irregular. Blood count may show eosinophilia. Treatment is with metronidazole.

Cow's milk protein intolerance

Allergy to cow's milk protein is rare and often over-diagnosed. The diarrhoea may be bloody, and urticaria, stridor, wheeze and very rarely Anaphylaxis can occur. It is less common in babies who have been breast-fed. Diagnosis is clinical, and symptoms should subside within a week of withdrawing cow's milk. The child should be rechallenged after a period of time (in hospital if original symptoms were severe). A hydrolysed protein formula milk should be used. In most cases intolerance resolves in 1–2 years.

Causes of recurrent abdominal pain

Idiopathic recurrent abdominal pain

Other
- Psychogenic
- Abdominal migraine
- Sickle cell disease

Hepatic
- ► Hepatitis

► Pancreas
- Pancreatitis

Gastrointestinal
- ► Irritable bowel syndrome
- Oesophagitis
- Peptic ulcer
- Inflammatory bowel disease
- ► Constipation
- Malabsorption
- Giardiasis

Gynaecological
- Dysmenorrhoea
- Pelvic inflammatory disease
- Haematocolpos
- Ovarian cyst

Urinary tract
- Infection

What you need from your evaluation

History

- Where is it worst ?(nonorganic pain is classically peri-umbilical)
- What time of day does it occur? (asking them to keep a diary may be useful)
- Does the pain affect daily activities? (school, sports, trips away)
- Are there constitutional symptoms such as weight loss, anorexia or fever?
- Are there gastrointestinal, urinary or gynaecological symptoms?
- Are there any emotional, anxiety or family problems?

Physical examination

- **Growth:** weight loss or fall-off in growth indicates serious pathology
- **General examination:** look for pallor, jaundice and clubbing
- **Abdominal examination:** is there hepatomegaly, splenomegaly, enlarged kidneys or a distended bladder?
- **Anorectal examination:** not routine in children

Investigations and their significance

Investigations are required only if your evaluation suggests an organic cause

• Full blood count	Anaemia, eosinophilia, infection (leucocytosis)
• CRP	Add stool test for H. pylori antigen (gastritis)
• Liver function tests	Liver dysfunction
• Urea and electrolytes	Renal failure
• Amylase	Pancreatitis
• Urinalysis and culture	Urine infection
• Stool for ova and parasites (3 samples)	GI parasites, e.g. giardiasis
• Occult blood	GI blood loss, e.g. inflammatory bowel disease or peptic ulcer
• Abdominal and pelvic ultrasound	Urinary obstruction at all levels, organomegaly, abscesses, pregnancy, ovarian cyst and torsion
• Plain abdominal radiograph	Constipation, renal calculi if radiopaque, lead poisoning
• Barium swallow and follow-through	Oesophagitis and reflux, peptic ulcer, Crohn's disease, congenital malformations of the gut
• Barium enema	Ulcerative colitis
• Endoscopy	Oesophagitis and reflux Peptic ulceration Inflammatory bowel disease

 Paediatrics at a Glance, Third Edition. Lawrence Miall, Mary Rudolf, Dominic Smith. © 2012 John Wiley & Sons, Ltd. Published 2012 by John Wiley & Sons, Ltd.

Some 10–15% of school-age children experience recurrent abdominal pain at some point, but only one in ten have an organic problem. A good clinical evaluation is essential as it is rare for organic problems to present with abdominal pain alone, although inflammatory bowel disease, chronic urine infections and parasites may do so.

Idiopathic recurrent abdominal pain

The majority of children presenting with recurrent abdominal pain have no identifiable organic cause. In this circumstance the expression 'recurrent abdominal pain' is often used as a diagnostic term in itself implying that the pain is functional rather than organic. The pain can be very real and severe. The periodicity of the complaint and the intervening good health are characteristic. The children are often described as being sensitive, anxious and high-achieving individuals, although this is by no means always true. Management must be directed towards reassurance, maximizing a normal lifestyle and minimizing school absence. (see box) In the majority of children the pain resolves over time.

Management of a child with recurrent abdominal pain

(These strategies may also be helpful for nonorganic headaches and leg 'growing' pains)

• Assure the parents and child that no major illness appears to be present.
• Explain that the aetiology is not known but nonetheless the pain is very real.
• Do not communicate to the parents that the child is malingering.
• Identify those symptoms and signs which the parents should watch for and which would suggest the need for a re-evaluation.
• Develop a system of return visits to monitor the symptom. Having the family keep a diary of pain episodes and related symptoms can be helpful.
• During return visits allow time for both the child and parent to express stresses and concerns.
• Make every effort to normalize the life of the child, encouraging attendance at school and participation in regular activities.
• Liaise with school to ensure consistent attendance.

Other causes

Psychogenic abdominal pain

In some children the abdominal pain is truly psychosomatic and related to stress at home or at school. Obviously these underlying causes must be addressed. In most cases simply indicating the link and explaining that children tend to experience tummy-aches in a similar way to how adults experience headaches is enough to reassure the parents and child. It is important to minimize absence from school.

Irritable bowel syndrome

This is a functional condition of the bowel associated with recurrent abdominal pain and minor GI symptoms such as bloating and altered bowel habit. There is sometimes alternating diarrhoea and constipation. Usually no psychological stresses are identified. There may be some overlap with "recurrent abdominal pain". It has been suggested that the discomfort results from a dysfunction of the autonomic system of the gut. The stool may be described as varying from pellets to unformed stool. Gas can also be a feature and many of these children give a history of colic as babies. IBS is a symptom based diagnosis (symptoms must be present for 6 months) and requires and organic cause to be excluded. It usually presents in young adults but can occur in children and teenagers. The acute symptoms resolve over time, but relapses are common. A change in symptoms (e.g. weight loss, bleeding or anaemia) should prompt further investigations and a re-evaluation of the diagnosis. Smooth muscle relaxants (e.g. mebeverine) may help abdominal spasms.

Gastritis and peptic ulcer

Gastritis and peptic ulcer are now recognized as an important cause of childhood abdominal pain. The features may be similar to adult ulcer symptoms—epigastric, relieved by food, and there may be a family history. If suspected a trial of an H_2-receptor antagonist, such as ranitidine, may be used empirically, but if symptoms are persistent investigations for *Helicobacter pylori* are indicated. These include stool examination for helicobacter antigen, hydrogen breath test, or endoscopy. Treatment consists of eradication with triple therapy (omeprazole, amoxicillin and metranidazole).

Parasitic infestations

The commonest GI parasite in the United Kingdom is *Giardia lamblia*. Inspection of the stool for presence of cysts or parasites (three separate samples are required) is merited in all children with recurrent abdominal pain. Threadworms do not cause pain, nor are they detectable on examination of the stool.

Other causes of recurrent abdominal pain

These include:
• Constipation (see Chapter 33)
• Inflammatory bowel disease (see Chapter 31)
• Urine infections (see Chapter 34)
• Sickle cell disease: Abdominal pain is a feature of sickle cell crisis (see Chapter 47- anaemia).

KEY POINTS

Nonorganic pain characteristically is:
• Periodic pain with intervening good health
• Often periumbilical
• May be related to school hours.

Consider organic pain if there is:
• Pain occurring at night
• Weight loss, reduced appetite, lack of energy, recurrent fever
• Organ-specific symptoms, e.g. change in bowel habit, polyuria, menstrual problems, vomiting, occult or frank bleeding
• Ill appearance, growth failure, swollen joints.

Causes of constipation

Acute causes

Fluid depletion
- Caused by fever or hot weather
- May require laxatives
- May lead to chronic constipation

▶ Bowel obstruction
- Rare and usually due to congenital gut malformation or adhesions following previous surgery
- Usually presents as acute abdomen, but may present as constipation with vomiting and abdominal pain

Signs that a child may be constipated
- Infrequent stools (<3 per week)
- Pain and straining on defecation
- Abdominal pain
- Small, hard stools
- Avoiding the toilet
- Not having an urge to defecate
- Difficulty finishing defecation
- Painful bottom
- Dribbling urine
- Faecal smell
- Leaking liquid stools into underwear

Chronic causes

▶ Functional constipation
- Common, particularly in disabled children
- Often stems from withholding from painful detaecation
- May cause megacolon
- Management involves laxatives, bowel training and diet
- Often recurs

▶ Hirschsprung's disease
- Onset in newborn period or infancy
- Failure to thrive and abdominal distension are features
- Diagnosis is by rectal biopsy

What you need from your evaluation

History
- Infrequent but normal stools are not indicators of constipation (although very long standing constipation can be painless)
- Ask about hardness of the stool, painful defecation, crampy abdominal pain and blood on the stool or toilet paper. History of an anal fissure is significant
- Onset in infancy suggests Hirschsprung's disease— functional constipation has a later onset
- Precipitating events include mismanagement of toilet training, and fluid depletion caused by hot weather, a febrile illness or vomiting
- Ask about diet as a basis for giving dietary advice on management of constipation
- Constipation can be a presenting feature of child maltreatment

Examination
- **Growth**
  Review the growth chart as Hirschsprung's disease is accompanied by failure to thrive

- **Abdominal examination**
  Hard indentable faeces are often palpated in the left lower quadrant

- **Anorectal examination**
  Rectal examination is not usually indicated, but will reveal hard stools. An anal fissure may be found on inspection of the anus

Investigations
- Plain abdominal radiograph is not usually required, but may show enormous quantities of faeces in the colon

- Hirschsprung's disease is diagnosed by rectal biopsy, and should be considered if constipation started in infancy and/or there is poor growth

- If there is growth faltering check for coeliac disease and hypothyroidism

Bristol Stool Chart

| Separate hard lumps, like nuts (hard to pass) | Sausage-shaped but lumpy | Like a sausage but with cracks on its surface | Like a sausage or snake, smooth and soft | Soft blobs with clear-cut edges (passed easily) | Fluffy pieces with ragged edges, a mushy stool | Watery, no solid pieces. Entirely liquid |

Management of constipation

Stage 1
• **Dietary management of constipation**
High-fibre foods
• Avoid excessive white bread
• Encourage wholewheat bread or bran
• High-fibre cereals
Stool softeners
• Fruit (particularly the peel), vegetables
• Beans and nuts
• Drink 6–8 glasses of water or juice per day
• Have a bottle of water available during school time
• Fluids of any sort, especially fresh orange or prune juice
• In babies, try boiled water or fresh orange juice between milk feeds

Stage 2: Disimpaction (for 1–2 weeks or until symptoms resolve)
• **Laxatives:**
  – **Iso-osmotic agents** such as polyethylene glycol (e.g. Movicol) carry water to the stool, softening and lubricating it. Increase the dose until the stools become liquid, then reduce,
  – **Stimulant laxatives** such as sodium picosulfate, bisacodyl, senna or ducosate sodium should be added if polyethylene glycol is ineffective.
  – **Osmotic laxatives** (e.g. lactulose) draw fluid into the bowel and can be used if polyethylene glycol is not tolerated.
• **Bulking agents:** absorb water and make stool softer (e.g. Fybogel).
• **Glycerin suppositories** are useful in babies.
• **Enemas:** may rarely be required in severe constipation if oral treatment has failed.
• **Manual evacuation under general anaesthetic:** occasionally required in extreme cases, usually in children with other problems such as severe learning difficulties.

Stage 3: Maintenance
• Stools should be kept soft by either diet (see box) or laxatives (polyethylene glycol ± stimulant)for 3–6 months.
• Encourage daily bowel movements by sitting the child on the toilet at a fixed time once or twice each day for 5–10 min. If done after eating this makes use of the gastrocolic reflex.

Stage 4: Vigilance
• Start or escalate treatment at the first indication of recurrence of hard stools.

In normal children the frequency of bowel movements ranges from more than two per day to none for several days. Infrequent bowel movements are common in exclusively breast-fed babies.

Constipation

Constipation is the infrequent passage of hard, pellet-like stools with excessive straining or painful defecation. Using the Bristol Stool Chart can help children describe what their stool is like. Infrequent but asymptomatic bowel movements alone do not constitute constipation. Chronic constipation is commonest aged 2–4 years when they are potty training. About a third of 4–7-year-olds are constipated at any given time. Constipation can have a sudden onset after an illness or if the child has not eaten or drunk well for a few days, or can develop insidiously.

• **Faecal impaction:** When there is no adequate bowel movement for days or weeks a large faecal mass can become compacted in the rectum.
• **Soiling** refers to faecal staining of the underwear and results from leakage of liquid stool around impacted faeces. It can be mistaken for diarrhoea. The term is also sometimes used when a child is delayed in gaining bowel control.
• **Encopresis** is the voluntary passage of whole formed stools in inappropriate places (including underwear) by a child who is mature enough to be continent. It is indicative of severe behavioural problems.

Idiopathic constipation
This often stems from painful passage of a hard stool which has caused an anal fissure. The child withholds further stools to avoid pain. Water is then reabsorbed from the colon making the stools harder and more painful to pass. The cycle becomes self-perpetuating and the rectum can become so stretched that colonic dilatation may occur (megacolon).

Prevention of constipation involves establishing a good toilet routine—toddlers and young children shouldn't be made to wait and shouldn't feel rushed when going to the toilet. Encourage exercise and a good diet (see box).

Management of established constipation involves checking for faecal impaction, evacuating the bowel, maintenance treatment and good diet (see boxes). Constipation often recurs, but is controllable with active management.

Hirschprung's disease
Hirschprung's disease (congenital aganglionosis) is the absence of ganglion cells in the bowel wall nerve plexus. It usually presents in the newborn period with delayed passage of meconium (for >48 hours after birth) and abdominal distension, but if only a short segment of bowel is affected it may present later with constipation and failure to thrive. It is much commoner in boys than girls. Various genes have been identified and there is an association with Down's syndrome. Diagnosis is made by barium enema and then rectal biopsy. Management is surgical with resection of the abnormal section of bowel.

Risk factors for constipation

Diet	Not drinking enough fluid or high fibre foods
Holding of stools	Unwillingness to use toilets (e.g. school or public toilets) or because they don't want to interrupt what they are doing
Change in routine	Going on holiday, moving house or school or even changing formula milk may upset bowel habit
Lack of exercise	Exercise can help with constipation. Lack of exercise makes it worse
Genetics	Sometimes a family history of constipation is present. Constipation is associated with various syndromes and with learning difficulties
Medication	Codeine, cough medicine, some anticonvulsants and antihistamines may cause constipation

Urinary tract infection

Urinary tract infections (UTIs) are common: they occur in 10% of girls and 3% of boys and 90% are due to infection with *Escherichia coli*. It is important to make a definite diagnosis as a UTI may indicate a congenital renal anomaly or vesicoureteric reflux, which if left untreated may lead to renal failure

Underlying causes of UTI

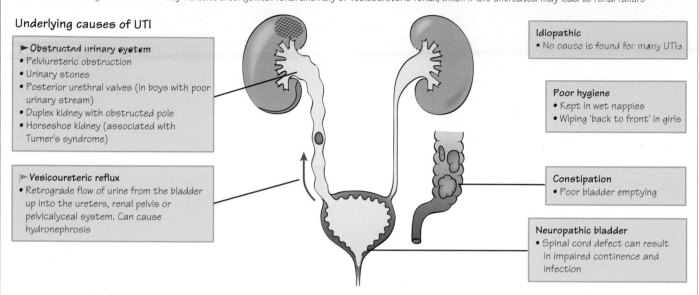

► Obstructed urinary system
- Pelviureteric obstruction
- Urinary stones
- Posterior urethral valves (in boys with poor urinary stream)
- Duplex kidney with obstructed pole
- Horseshoe kidney (associated with Turner's syndrome)

► Vesicoureteric reflux
- Retrograde flow of urine from the bladder up into the ureters, renal pelvis or pelvicalyceal system. Can cause hydronephrosis

Idiopathic
- No cause is found for many UTIs

Poor hygiene
- Kept in wet nappies
- Wiping 'back to front' in girls

Constipation
- Poor bladder emptying

Neuropathic bladder
- Spinal cord defect can result in impaired continence and infection

What you need from your evaluation

History

- Antenatal ultrasound (anomaly scans can detect structural urinary
- tract problems)
- In infancy UTI can present with fever, vomiting, irritability, septic shock, poor feeding, failure to thrive, jaundice
- Poor force of urinary stream can be a sign of posterior urethral valves in infant boys
- In older children UTI can present with fever, abdominal pain, dysuria, bedwetting, haematuria, offensive smelling urine
- Risk factors for UTI; constipation, dehydration, spinal disorders
- Review family history for vesico-ureteric reflux or other renal disease

Examination

- Signs of general illness – fever, perfusion, pulse rate, jaundice
- Abdominal pain, palpable kidneys or bladder
- Growth measurement and blood pressure
- Spinal abnormalities and peripheral nervous system
- Genitalia

Treatment

- Young infants < 3 months are admitted and started on intravenous antibiotics such as cefotaxime or gentamicin
- Children with pyelonephritis signs are admitted and treated with intravenous antibiotic for 2-4 days followed by a course of oral antibiotics to 10 days
- Children with UTI without pyelonephritis can usually be managed in the community with oral antibiotic for 3 days (e.g trimotheprim, nitrofurantoin, cephalosporin)
- Longer term prophylactic oral antibiotic is considered for infants and children with recurrent UTI or suspected vesicoureteric reflux
- Longer term strategies are advised to ensure good hygiene, adequate fluid intake, and prompt toileting to reduce delay in voiding

Investigations

- Urine analysis is vital to confirm infection but samples can easily be contaminated by bacteria on the skin around the genitalia
- Urine collection by clean catch if possible
- Urine bag or pad sample if clean catch not possible
- Urine should reach laboratory within 4 hours or be stored in fridge or boric acid container
- Presence of infection suggested by
  - MC&S - Microscopy (> 50 white cells per high power field, bacteria seen)
    - Culture (>100 000 colony forming bacterial units), checks sensitivity to antibiotic
  - Urinalysis by dipstick testing for leucocyte esterase, nitrites, blood
  Note white cells can be present in urine without infection in febrile children
- Imaging

Key points

- UTIs are common, especially in girls
- Fever may be the only symptom in infants
- Always confirm infection by culture
- Confirmed UTIs require investigation in all children
- In infancy check for obstruction and reflux

 Paediatrics at a Glance, Third Edition. Lawrence Miall, Mary Rudolf, Dominic Smith. © 2012 John Wiley & Sons, Ltd. Published 2012 by John Wiley & Sons, Ltd.

Investigating urinary tract infections

Renal ultrasound scan (USS)	To identify anatomical abnormalities (e.g. hydronephrosis, gross vesicoureteric reflux (VUR), duplex or horseshoe kidney). May identify renal cortical damage but can miss minor scarring
DMSA isotope scan	Injection of radioisotope that is taken up by the renal tubule and measured using a gamma camera. Used to quantify differential function between the two kidneys and show areas of scarring
DTPA or MAG-3 renogram	Injection of radioisotope that is filtered through renal tubule. Shows functional clearance and can identify stasis of urine in the renal pelvis due to obstruction
Micturating cystourethrogram (MCUG)	A catheter is passed into the bladder and contrast injected to detect reflux up into the ureters with antibiotic cover

In most cases the urinary tract infection (UTI) occurs in a child with a normal renal tract and does not cause any lasting damage. In one third of cases there may be an anatomical congenital abnormality which predisposes to UTI by causing stasis of urine in an obstructed or refluxing urinary system (vesicoureteric reflux). Recurrent urinary infections can cause renal parenchymal scarring which may lead to complications of hypertension and renal impairment. This can occasionally cause end-stage renal failure. For this reason there are recommendations regarding investigation of children with UTI:

Initial management
- **Child <3 months with signs of any sepsis:** investigate with full septic screen including urine sample for microscopy, culture and sensitivities (MC&S) and treat with IV antibiotics
- **Child 3 months to 3 years with signs of possible UTI:** send urine sample MC&S and start antibiotics
- **Child >3 years with possible UTI:**
- Use urine dipstick analysis:
  - nitrite (+) = probable UTI, send urine MC&S and start antibiotic
  - leucocyte (+) but nitrite (–) = equivocal, send urine MC&S
- Do not start antibiotic unless good clinical evidence of UTI
- Both leucocyte (–) and nitrite (–) = negative, do not send for culture, do not start antibiotics.

Further investigation
Further investigation for anatomical problems and scarring depends on the child's age and whether there are clinical features of more severe, recurrent or atypical infection. The aim is to screen children at higher risk of VUR.

The level of further imaging depends on the child's age and severity of symptoms. A young baby with UTI is at high risk of reflux and should have full imaging with USS DMSA and MCUG. An older child with mild symptoms in whom infection responds quickly to antibiotics may need no further imaging.

Renal anomalies
Congenital renal anomalies are common (8/1000 live births). Less than 5% of these will have long-term renal impairment.
- **Solitary kidney:** A single kidney due to unilateral renal agenesis.
- **Ectopic kidney:** Abnormal migration during embryogenesis leads to a pelvic or horseshoe kidney.
- **Multicystic dysplastic kidney:** The kidney is non-functioning and usually involutes and disappears by school age.
- **Autosomal dominant polycystic kidney disease (ADPKD):** Occurs in 1 in 1000 children and adults. Small cysts are present throughout the kidney. The enlarged kidneys may cause haematuria, hypertension and renal failure later in adult life.
- **Autosomal recessive polycystic kidney disease (ARPKD):** This rare condition (1 in 20 000) is often diagnosed antenatally as the large, cystic kidneys do not produce adequate urine, leading to reduced amniotic fluid and secondary pulmonary hypoplasia. If the child survives the neonatal period they develop end-stage renal failure early in childhood.

Urological abnormalities
Obstructive uropathy may be due to an obstruction at the level of the renal pelvis, the junction of the ureter with the bladder or at the bladder outlet. Obstructive uropathy can predispose to UTI and if severe can lead to renal impairment or failure.
- **Pelviureteric obstruction** is due to abnormal tissue or external compression at the point the renal pelvis joins the ureter. 75% improve without the need for surgical intervention.
- **Posterior urethral valves** occurs in 1 in 10 000 male infants. It is due to persistence of an embryological fold across the urethra, causing bladder hypertrophy, bilateral hydronephrosis and renal impairment.
- **Hypospadias:** The external urinary meatus opens on the ventral side of the penis. It may be mild, needing no treatment, or severe, requiring surgical repair. For this reason parents should be advised not to have the child circumcised, so that the foreskin tissue can be used in reconstructive surgery.
- **Phimosis:** The foreskin is non-retractile. This is normal in infancy and requires surgery only if there is an obstruction problem.
- **Paraphimosis:** The foreskin becomes trapped behind the glans causing pain and swelling. It is usually reducible without surgery.

  Circumcision is most commonly performed for persistence of these problems, or for cultural or religious reasons.

Vesicoureteric reflux
The retrograde flow of urine from the bladder into the ureters can cause hydronephrosis and predispose to UTI, pyelonephritis, hypertension or end-stage renal failure. VUR occurs because of an abnormally short and straight insertion of the ureters through the wall of the bladder, so that they are not properly occluded during bladder contraction. The severity of VUR is graded depending on extent of reflux and degree of dilatation of ureters, renal pelvis and calyces. VUR can be managed with conservative treatment (surveillance monitoring and antibiotics for infection). Around 50% resolve but surgery may be needed if there are breakthrough infections or deteriorating renal function.

Haematuria and proteinuria

Causes of haematuria

Post-streptococcal glomerulonephritis
- Preceding throat or skin infection
- Microscopic +/- macroscopic haematuria
- Red cells, casts, protein in urine
- Reduced renal function
- Hypertension

Polycystic kidneys
- Enlarged cystic kidneys
- Autosomal recessive form—infancy
- Autosomal dominant—adolescence

Renal stone
- Colicky pain

Other causes
- Henoch–Schönlein purpura (See Chapter 53)
- Thin basement membrane disease
- Kidney stone
- Kidney tumour
- Trauma
- Sickle cell disease
- Alport's syndrome
- IgA nephropathy

Renal tumour
- Abdominal mass
- Abdominal pain

Sickle cell disease

Renal trauma

Urinary tract infection
- Fever, vomiting, dysuria
- Urine dipstick test nitrites & leucocytes
- Urine culture positive

Causes of proteinuria

Nephrotic syndrome
- Oedema (facial puffiness, limb and scrotal oedema)
- Hypoalbuminaemia with ascites and pleural effusions
- Hyperlipidaemia
- Usually 'minimal change' glomerulonephritis
- Commonly relapses

Acute renal failure
(haematuria and proteinuria)

Orthostatic proteinuria
- After exercise or standing

Urinary tract infection
- With leucocytes and haematuria

What you need from your evaluation

History

Haematuria
- Make sure you are clear what is being described: is it frank blood, pink urine or a positive dipstick test. (Dipsticks are extremely sensitive to the presence of tiny quantities of blood)
- What colour is the urine? Brown suggests renal origin; fresh red blood or clots suggest bladder origin. Red urine can also be caused by eating beetroot or taking rifampicin
- Are there any other urinary symptoms? Frequency and dysuria suggest a UTI
- Is there severe pain? Renal colic or abdominal pain suggests a calculus (stone) or other obstruction
- Was there a precipitating factor? Enquire about trauma to the kidneys. Throat infections or skin infections may precede acute glomerulonephritis, or nephrotic syndrome and intense exercise may precipitate haematuria
- Is there a family history of renal disease or deafness? (Alport's syndrome causes deafness and nephritis, and is autosomal dominant)

Investigations and their significance

- Urinalysis and culture — For presence of blood, protein, casts or white cells. Pyuria and bactiuria point to a UTI
- Full blood count — For anaemia and to exclude HUS
- ASOT/throat swab — For evidence of streptococcal infection
- U&E — To assess renal function
- Serum C3 complement level — Will be low in some types of glomerulonephritis
- Serum albumin level — Low in nephrotic syndrome
- Urinary protein/creatinine ratio — High in nephrotic syndrome
- Triglycerides and cholesterol level — High in nephrotic syndrome
- Renal ultrasound and AXR — May show renal stones
- Renal biopsy — If renal function impaired or if there is hypertension, proteinuria and haematuria

Nephrotic syndrome
- Has oedema around the eyes been noticed in the morning? Has there been any weight gain?
- What is the urine output? Is the child fluid restricted to a certain volume per day?
- Is this the first presentation or a relapse?
- If the latter, what has the child been treated with in the past?

Examination

- Blood pressure measurement is mandatory. Hypertension suggests renal disease
- Palpate the abdomen for renal masses (tumour, polycystic kidneys or obstruction) and check for ascites
- Check for pitting oedema over the tibia and sacrum
- Examine for the presence of pleural effusions
- Measure weight and compare with previous values
- Look for any purpuric rash (Henoch–Schönlein purpura (p. 101) or haemolytic uraemic syndrome, HUS)

Acute post-streptococcal glomerulonephritis

Acute glomerulonephritis results from immune-mediated damage to the glomerulus. The commonest type in childhood is due to immune complex formation following group A beta-haemolytic streptococcal infection. The presenting complaint is usually haematuria, which is cola coloured and typically occurs 1–2 weeks after a throat or 3–6 weeks after a skin infection. The child may have malaise, oedema, loin pain and headache or be asymptomatic. Urinalysis shows gross haematuria with granular and red cell casts and often proteinuria. In most children there is mild oliguria (reduced urine output) but in a minority there may be acute renal failure and hypertension. Useful investigations include a throat swab and antistreptolysin O (ASO) titre to look for evidence of streptococcal infection and there may be a low C3 complement level.

A 10-day course of penicillin is recommended to try to clear the nephritic strain of streptococcus, although there is no evidence that this alters the course of the disease. Acute renal failure is managed with careful monitoring of fluid balance and renal function. Salt and fluid restriction may be required and hypertension must be controlled. Rarely, acute glomerulonephritis leads to severe renal failure requiring renal dialysis.

Nephrotic syndrome

Nephrotic syndrome is characterized by proteinuria, low albumin, oedema and high triglycerides. This is due to increased capillary wall permeability in the glomerulus which allows protein to leak into the urine. The commonest cause (85%) is 'minimal change' glomerulonephritis (MCGN), where the histological changes on renal biopsy are very mild. This type usually responds to steroid therapy. The presenting feature is oedema, which is usually most noticeable in the mornings around the eyelids and as pitting oedema on the legs. There may be history of a recent viral upper respiratory tract infection (URTI). Focal segmental glomerulosclerosis (FSGS) is the second most frequent form.

With time, weight gain, ascites and pleural effusions develop secondary to the hypoalbuminaemia. Hypertension is rare, but there may be anorexia, abdominal pain, diarrhoea and oliguria. There is an increased risk of infection due to leakage of immunoglobulins, and an increased risk of thrombosis. Urinalysis shows excessive protein and there is low serum albumin, high triglyceride and cholesterol levels and normal C3 complement.

Treatment of minimal change nephrotic syndrome involves fluid restriction, a low salt diet and corticosteroids (prednisolone). Prednisolone is continued until there is remission of proteinuria, continued at a weaning dose over 2–3 months. Parents should be warned about the immunosuppressive effects of nephrotic syndrome and steroids and should avoid live vaccines and chickenpox at this time. Prophylactic penicillin is given until the proteinuria has cleared.

Relapses are common, occurring in up to 75% of those who initially respond. Children who are steroid resistant need a renal biopsy to confirm the pathology and may need treatment with cyclophosphamide. Long-term prognosis is good although delayed relapses may occur. Other forms of nephrotic syndrome (e.g. following Henoch–Schönlein purpura) carry a worse prognosis and may progress to chronic renal failure requiring dialysis and eventually transplantation.

Other renal conditions
Acute renal failure

Acute renal failure is defined as a rapid onset of anuria or severe oliguria (<0.5 mL/kg per hour). Causes can be divided into prerenal (i.e. poor perfusion), renal or postrenal (due to urinary obstruction). The commonest prerenal cause is hypovolaemic shock. Prerenal failure can usually be managed with fluid replacement and inotropic support of the circulation.

Intrinsic renal causes include the following:
- Acute tubular necrosis (often secondary to shock)
- Haemolytic uraemic syndrome (HUS)
- Vasculitis and glomerulonephritis
- Renal vein thrombosis
- Nephrotoxic drugs (e.g. gentamicin, vancomycin).

Renal failure requires careful inpatient management. Hyperkalaemia, hypertension and fluid overload can be life-threatening complications. If conservative management is failing, there is severe electrolyte imbalance, progressive acidosis or fluid overload, and renal dialysis is then necessary, via peritoneal dialysis or haemodialysis.

Haemolytic uraemic syndrome

Haemolytic uraemic syndrome (HUS) is an important cause of renal failure associated with thrombocytopenia, renal failure and haemolytic anaemia due to fragmentation of red blood cells. It often follows an episode of bloody diarrhoea and is associated with a verotoxin producing *E. coli* O157:H7. The disease can also affect the brain, causing encephalopathy. Intensive care treatment may be needed for renal failure, encephalopathy and associated colitis. Chronic renal failure can result.

Chronic renal failure

Approximately 1000 children in the UK receive renal replacement therapy. The commonest cause is a congenital structural renal abnormality such as 'cystic–dysplastic' kidneys or severe obstructive nephropathy. Rarer causes include glomerulonephritis and renal disease as part of autoimmune systemic disease. Children with untreated chronic renal failure are at risk of anaemia, difficulty with exertion, poor appetite, poor growth, osteodystrophy and hypertension.

Management involves a high-calorie, low-protein diet that is low in phosphate. Growth hormone and vitamin D supplements are often required and anaemia may be treated with erythropoietin injections. When the renal disease becomes end stage, children require dialysis. Dialysis can either be haemodialysis (in hospital) or peritoneal dialysis (can be administered at home). The best long-term treatment is renal transplant from a cadaveric or living related donor.

KEY POINTS

- Careful urine analysis is essential.
- Haematuria is more likely to have serious underlying cause if associated with hypertension, proteinuria, impaired function.
- Nephrotic syndrome usually responds to steroid treatment but relapses may occur.
- Renal transplantation is the treatment of choice for end-stage renal disease.

Bedwetting and daytime wetting

Nocturnal enuresis refers to bedwetting. It usually occurs in normal children and is due to a delay in the development of the normal sphincter control mechanisms. Day and night wetting (diurnal enuresis) may be due to poor bladder sensation or bladder muscle instability. Secondary enuresis refers to wetting in a child who had previously been dry, and is often associated with psychological stress

► **Primary nocturnal enuresis**
- Common: 10% of 5-year-olds and 3% of 12-year-olds wet the bed once a week
- As in familial. Twice as common in boys than girls

Causes
- Delayed maturation (often familial)
- May be reduced ADH production
- Reduced bladder awareness
- Emotional stress
- Urinary tract infection
- Polyuria due to diabetes or renal disease

Causes of secondary enuresis
- Emotional upset
- ► Urinary tract infection
- Diabetes mellitus
- Threadworm infection

Causes of diurnal enuresis
- Urinary tract infection
- Neurogenic bladder
- Congenital abnormality (e.g. ectopic ureter)
- Severe constipation
- Psychogenic, due to stress
- ► Sexual abuse
- Physiological (urgency)

What you need from your evaluation

History
- Has the child ever been dry? If so, at what age? Was there a particular trigger that led to wetting again (e.g. birth of a sibling)?
- Is there a family history of primary nocturnal enuresis? Ask about siblings, parents and grandparents
- Is there anything to suggest stress as a cause? Is there any possibility of sexual abuse?
- Is there any dysuria, frequency or systemic upset to suggest a urinary tract infection? Is the child constipated?
- Has there been a sudden onset of polyuria, polydipsia, or weight loss to suggest diabetes mellitus or other renal disease?
- How have the parents dealt with the wetting? Have they punished or criticized the child for wetting in the past? Do they have false expectations?
- What methods have they tried, e.g. fluid restriction, lifting onto the toilet at night, star charts?
- What is the pattern of the wetting—nocturnal only, day and night, with urgency or with dribbling incontinence? Are there any features in the history to suggest a neuropathic bladder?

Examination
- Is there any evidence of a neurological or congenital abnormality? Check leg reflexes and perineal sensation.
- Look for evidence of spina bifida occulta such as a lipoma or hairy patch over the sacral area
- Is there a palpable faecal mass (constipation)?
- Is there evidence of renal disease?
- Check for hypertension

Investigations and their significance
- Urine microscopy and culture — To exclude UTI
- Urine dipstick — To exclude glycosuria
- Renal ultrasound and isotope scan, — If ectopic ureter strongly suspected. (This causes a constant connection to the vagina rather than the bladder)

Key points
- Enuresis is common—15% of 5-year-olds wet the bed
- There is rarely an organic cause
- The majority respond to behavioural management
- Psychological stress should be considered in secondary enuresis

Management of primary nocturnal enuresis
- Intervention is not usually advised until the age of 7 years or more, when the child can take some responsibility and normal sphincter control has developed
- Behavioural management with star charts and rewards for dry nights is helpful
- An enuresis alarm, which wakes children when they start to urinate so that they learn to wake up and go to the toilet, is often the most effective treatment and works within a few weeks
- Bladder training—allow unrestricted drinking during the day to 'teach' the child to tolerate a full bladder
- Avoid caffeinated drinks and fruit juice. Do not overly restrict fluid intake. Lifting is best avoided as it trains the child to void whilst half asleep Desmopressin (antidiuretic hormone) can be given by nasal spray or tablets at night. This reduces urine output and can be particularly useful for short periods such as going on camp or staying with friends. Oxybutynin reduces detrusor muscle instability in children with a small bladder capacity and urgency
- Treat any constipation

Swellings in the groin and scrotum and impalpable testes

Inguinal hernia
- Common in preterm infants
- Often increases in size when the child is crying
- Swelling extends up into the groin, does not transilluminate
- Testis is palpable, distinct from the swelling
- Reduction of the swelling is diagnostic
- No pain unless incarcerated
- Requires surgery

Inguinal lymphadenopathy
- Firm nodules with clear borders
- May be tender
- Responsible infected lesion may be found on the leg

► Testicular torsion
- Tender swollen scrotum
- Intense pain
- Occurs in pubertal boys
- Requires urgent surgery

► Hydrocele
- Often present from birth and usually resolves by 12 months
- No pain
- Does not extend into the groin
- Testis cannot be palpated through the fluid
- Transilluminates

Impalpable testes

► Retractile testis
- Brought down by careful palpation
- Examine the child with warm hands, and cross-legged or squatting

Undescended testis
- May be unilateral or bilateral
- More common in premature babies
- 5% undescended at term, 1% by 12 months
- May be associated with inguinal hernia
- Orchidopexy required by 1 year to avoid infertility, torsion and malignancy
- Bilateral impalpable testes need very careful evaluation (see below)

Ectopic testes
- Testes descend but along abnormal path
- May be in superficial inguinal pouch or on perineum

What you need from your evaluation

History

- **Characteristics of the swelling:** an incarcerated hernia and testicular torsion are both painful. Hernias usually cause intermittent swelling. Hydroceles are often present from birth

Key points

- Incarcerated inguinal hernia and testicular torsion are emergencies
- Hydroceles are present from birth and usually resolve spontaneously
- Undescended testes must be referred by 1 year of age

Physical examination

For a swelling
- **Observation:** is the boy in pain? Does the swelling extend into the groin?
- **Palpation:** in an inguinal hernia the swelling extends right up into the groin, and the testis is palpable separate from the swelling. In a hydrocele the testis cannot be palpated through the fluid. Testicular torsion is acutely tender
- Bilateral inguinal hernias in a girl should raise the possibility of the swellings being testes in an undervirilized male with ambiguous genitalia
- Bilateral impalpable testes may rarely be the manifestation of a virilized female (e.g. congenital adrenal hyperplasia or other disorders of sexual
- differentiation) A pelvic ultrasound should be performed urgently
- Impalpable testes can be a sign of severe anterior pituitary dysfunction, especially if associated with micro-penis
  Reduction of the swelling by manipulation or spontaneously is diagnostic of a hernia
  Transillumination: when a torch is held to the scrotum a hydrocele transilluminates but a hernia does not
  General examination: if lymphadenopathy is suspected as a cause, look for an infected lesion on the leg, lymphadenopathy elsewhere, and check for hepatosplenomegaly

Causes of developmental delay

Idiopathic
- Autism
- Various dysmorphic syndromes

Chromosomal abnormalities
- Down's syndrome
- Fragile X

Perinatal injury
- Asphyxia
- Birth trauma

Prenatal injury
- Fetal alcohol syndrome
- Intrauterine infections (TORCH)

Endocrine and metabolic defects
- Congenital hypothyroidism
- Phenylketonuria

Neurodegenerative disorders
- Leucomalacia

Neurocutaneous syndromes
- Sturge–Weber
- Neurofibromatosis
- Tuberous sclerosis

Postnatal injury
- Meningitis
- Non-accidental injury
- Neglect

Central nervous system malformation
- Neural tube defects
- Hydrocephalus

What you need from your evaluation

History

Developmental milestones
- Enquire systematically about milestones for the four developmental areas
- Ascertain the extent of delay and which areas are affected
- Remember to allow for prematurity during the first 2 years. Beyond that catch-up in development rarely occurs
- Loss in skills suggests a neurodegenerative condition
- Ask whether there are concerns about vision and hearing

Past medical history
- Enquire into alcohol consumption, medical problems and medication during pregnancy
- Enquire about prematurity and neonatal complications

Family history
- Ask about learning difficulties and consanguinity

Physical examination

Children are often uncooperative so parental report is particularly important

Developmental skills
- Assess each developmental area in turn: gross motor, fine motor/adaptive, language and social skills
- Attempt to evaluate vision and hearing
- Assess factors such as alertness, responsiveness, interest in surroundings, determination and concentration; these all have positive influences on a child's attainments

General examination
- Dysmorphic signs suggest a genetic defect, chromosome anomaly or teratogenic effect
- Microcephaly at birth suggests fetal alcohol syndrome or intrauterine infections
- Poor growth is common, but may be due to hypothyroidism or non-organic failure to thrive (look for signs of neglect)
- Look for café-au-lait spots, depigmented patches and portwine stains which are indicative of neurocutaneous syndromes
- Hepatosplenomegaly suggests a metabolic disorder

Neurological examination
- Look for abnormalities in tone, strength and coordination, deep tendon reflexes, clonus, cranial nerves and primitive reflexes, and ocular abnormalities

Investigations

- Chromosome analysis, thyroid function tests and urine screen for metabolic defects are usually obtained in global developmental delay
- More sophisticated metabolic investigations and brain imaging may be indicated for some
- A hearing test is mandatory in language delay

The term *global* developmental delay refers to delay in all milestones (but particularly language, fine motor and social skills) and is particularly worrying as it generally indicates significant learning disability. Delay in a single area is much less concerning. Warning signs suggesting significant developmental problems are described in the table on p. 20, Chapter 3.

You may need to repeat assessments to get an accurate view of a child's difficulties, and may need to refer on to an appropriate therapist for further assessment and guidance. When developmental difficulties are complex, the child should be seen by a Child Development Team (Chapter 42) for assessment and therapy. It is essential that parents' concerns are properly addressed. Ongoing parental anxiety in itself can be damaging to the child.

Severe learning disabilities (mental retardation)

The commonest causes of severe learning disability are Down's syndrome (Chapter 63), fragile X (Chapter 63) and cerebral palsy (Chapter 42). As the field of genetics advances, and genetic databases have been developed, more diagnoses are being made, particularly in children with congenital anomalies and dysmorphic features. It is therefore worth taking blood for genetic analysis. However, more than one third of children with global developmental delay still have no specific diagnosis.

Intrauterine infections

Primary infection with rubella, cytomegalovirus (CMV) or toxoplasmosis during early pregnancy can cause severe fetal damage, leading to multiple handicaps and microcephaly. Visual and hearing deficits are common.

Fetal alcohol syndrome

The fetal alcohol syndrome is a common cause of learning disabilities. It is caused by a moderate to high intake of alcohol during pregnancy. Children have a characteristic facial appearance, cardiac defects, poor growth and microcephaly. The severity of the problems relate to the quantity of alcohol consumed.

Congenital hypothyroidism

Lack of thyroid hormone in the first years of life has a devastating effect on both growth and development. However, since neonatal screening has been introduced, it is now a rare cause of developmental delay. The defect is due to abnormal development of the thyroid or inborn errors of thyroxine metabolism.

Babies usually look normal at birth, but may show features of severe hypothyroidism (once called cretinism), including coarse facial features, hypotonia, a large tongue, an umbilical hernia, constipation, prolonged jaundice and a hoarse cry. Older babies or children have delayed development, lethargy and short stature. Thyroid function tests reveal low T4 and high TSH levels.

Congenital hypothyroidism is one of the few treatable causes of learning disabilities. Thyroid replacement is needed lifelong and must be monitored carefully as the child grows. If therapy is started in the first few weeks of life and compliance is good, normal growth and development can be achieved.

Inborn errors of metabolism

This group of disorders are caused by single-gene mutations, inherited in an autosomal recessive manner, so consanguinity is common. They present in a variety of ways of which developmental delay is one, but neonatal seizures, hypoglycaemia, vomiting and coma may also occur. Children sometimes have coarse features, microcephaly, failure to thrive and hepatosplenomegaly. These inborn errors of metabolism are rare; phenylketonuria is the commonest and is routinely screened for in all neonates.

Neurodegenerative disorders

A neurodegenerative disease is characterized by progressive deterioration of neurological function. The causes are heterogeneous and include biochemical defects, chronic viral infections and toxic substances, although many remain without an identified cause. Children may have coarse features, fits and intellectual deterioration, and microcephaly. The course is generally one of relentless and inevitable neurological deterioration, although bone marrow transplantation is now providing hope in some conditions

Neurocutaneous syndromes

The neurocutaneous syndromes are a heterogeneous group of disorders characterized by neurological dysfunction and skin lesions. In some individuals there may be severe learning disabilities and in others intelligence is normal. Examples include Sturge–Weber syndrome, neurofibromatosis and tuberous sclerosis. The aetiology of these problems is not known, but most are familial.

Abuse and neglect

Emotional abuse and neglect can have serious consequences for a child's developmental progress. The delay is often associated with failure to thrive. On presentation the child may be apathetic, look physically neglected with dirty clothing, unkempt hair and nappy rash, and there may be signs of non-accidental injury. If there is any suggestion of regression of developmental skills, chronic subdural haematomas (which can occur as a result of shaking injuries) should be considered.

Intensive input and support is needed. Day nurseries can provide good stimulation, nutrition and care. If children continue to be at risk for ongoing abuse or neglect they must be removed from the home. The prognosis depends on the degree of the damage incurred and how early the intervention is provided. Children who require removal from the home often have irreversible learning and emotional difficulties.

> ## KEY POINTS
>
> - All developmental areas must be accurately assessed in turn.
> - Remember to correct for prematurity in the first 2 years, and carry out a full physical and neurological examination.
> - Repeat evaluations may be required over time.
> - Attempt to make a diagnosis or identify the aetiology for the difficulties.
> - Involve the Child Development Team if difficulties are complex.

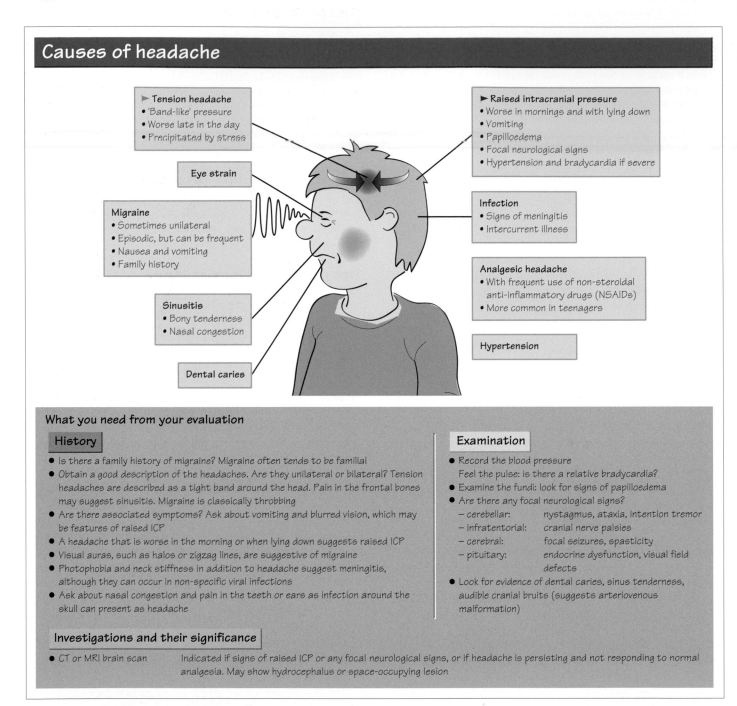

Causes of headache

▶ Tension headache
- 'Band-like' pressure
- Worse late in the day
- Precipitated by stress

Eye strain

Migraine
- Sometimes unilateral
- Episodic, but can be frequent
- Nausea and vomiting
- Family history

Sinusitis
- Bony tenderness
- Nasal congestion

Dental caries

▶ Raised intracranial pressure
- Worse in mornings and with lying down
- Vomiting
- Papilloedema
- Focal neurological signs
- Hypertension and bradycardia if severe

Infection
- Signs of meningitis
- Intercurrent illness

Analgesic headache
- With frequent use of non-steroidal anti-inflammatory drugs (NSAIDs)
- More common in teenagers

Hypertension

What you need from your evaluation

History

- Is there a family history of migraine? Migraine often tends to be familial
- Obtain a good description of the headaches. Are they unilateral or bilateral? Tension headaches are described as a tight band around the head. Pain in the frontal bones may suggest sinusitis. Migraine is classically throbbing
- Are there associated symptoms? Ask about vomiting and blurred vision, which may be features of raised ICP
- A headache that is worse in the morning or when lying down suggests raised ICP
- Visual auras, such as halos or zigzag lines, are suggestive of migraine
- Photophobia and neck stiffness in addition to headache suggest meningitis, although they can occur in non-specific viral infections
- Ask about nasal congestion and pain in the teeth or ears as infection around the skull can present as headache

Examination

- Record the blood pressure
  Feel the pulse: is there a relative bradycardia?
- Examine the fundi: look for signs of papilloedema
- Are there any focal neurological signs?
  - cerebellar: nystagmus, ataxia, intention tremor
  - infratentorial: cranial nerve palsies
  - cerebral: focal seizures, spasticity
  - pituitary: endocrine dysfunction, visual field defects
- Look for evidence of dental caries, sinus tenderness, audible cranial bruits (suggests arteriovenous malformation)

Investigations and their significance

- CT or MRI brain scan — Indicated if signs of raised ICP or any focal neurological signs, or if headache is persisting and not responding to normal analgesia. May show hydrocephalus or space-occupying lesion

Headaches are a common complaint in older children and are nearly always due to non-specific viral infection, local infection (e.g. sinusitis) or related to tension. Most pathological and serious headaches due to raised intracranial pressure can usually be differentiated clinically. If a headache is acute and severe, and the child is ill, then serious pathology such as intracranial infection, meningitis, haemorrhage or tumour must be considered. The following are features which should cause concern:
- Acute onset of severe pain
- Worse on lying down
- Associated vomiting
- Developmental regression or personality change

- Unilateral pain
- Hypertension
- Papilloedema
- Increasing head circumference
- Focal neurological signs.

Migraine

This is a common condition in school-age children and is slightly commoner in boys than girls. It is thought to result from constriction followed by dilatation and pulsation of intracranial arteries. Onset is usually in late childhood or early adolescence. Classically the attack starts with an aura such as 'zigzag' vision, followed by a throbbing unilateral headache with nausea and vomiting, although only 20% describe a preceding aura. Sleep usually ends the attack. In younger children the headache may be bilateral with no preceding aura and no vomiting. Parents often describe the child going very pale. Migraines always cause some reduction in the child's ability to function normally during the attack. There is no diagnostic test and physical examination is normal. The diagnosis is made clinically on the basis of the following.
- Episodic occurrence of headache (rarely every day, but can occur several times a week)
- Completely well between attacks
- Aura (often visual), though aura is less common in childhood (20%)
- Nausea in 90% of cases, sometimes vomiting
- Throbbing headache, sometimes unilateral
- Positive family history, usually in the mother
- Impairment of normal function during an attack
- Attack lasts between 1 and 72 hours.

The first line treatment is rest and simple analgesia. Combination therapy containing paracetamol and anti-emetics may be useful. Sleep deprivation and stress can predispose to migraine. Avoiding cheese, chocolate, citrus fruits, nuts and caffeinated drinks may be helpful. Ask the child to keep a migraine diary so you can identify triggers. Very frequent or severe attacks may warrant prophylaxis with beta-blockers or pizotifen. Migraine often persists into adulthood, but spontaneous remission does occur. In adolescents serotonin agonists (e.g. sumitriptan) can be given during an acute attack. Migraine can occasionally cause a post-migraine third nerve palsy or hemiparesis, though more serious cerebrovascular causes must always be excluded if this occurs.

Tension headache

Tension headaches are common in older school-age children. They may be due to contraction of neck or temporal muscles and are felt as a constricting band-like ache, which is usually worse towards the end of the day but does not interfere with sleep. The cause is often difficult to identify, but a proportion of children will be under some stress, either at home or school. Other family members may suffer similar headaches. Physical examination is normal. Management involves reassurance that there is no serious pathology, rest, sympathy and simple analgesia. Any underlying stress or anxiety in the child's life should be addressed. School absence should be minimized, and the school may need to be involved in developing a management strategy for when the headaches occur.

Tension headaches usually become less frequent or resolve spontaneously as the child gets older.

Cluster headache

These may occur in older children. There is sudden onset of very severe unilateral periorbital pain. Attacks occur in clusters a few times a day for a period of weeks. The pain is non-pulsatile and can occur at night as well as during the day and is exacerbated by alcohol. There may be unilateral eye redness, orbital swelling or tears. The cause may be due to neurotransmitter activity around the superficial temporal artery. Sumitriptan, a serotonin agonist, can be used acutely and calcium channel blockers (e.g. nifedipine) may help in recurrent attacks.

Raised intracranial pressure

Brain tumours, subdural haematomas and abscesses are all rare causes of headache in children. Anxiety about brain tumours is common amongst parents, though these rarely present with headache alone. If a headache is particularly persistent then neuroimaging may be required to put everyone's mind at rest. If neurological signs (e.g. nerve palsy or weakness) are detected then neuroimaging is mandatory.

Headaches due to raised intracranial pressure are classically worse on lying down and worse in the mornings, and may wake the child from sleep. There may be associated vomiting, often with surprisingly little nausea. Raised intracranial pressure may also cause blurred vision, high blood pressure and focal nerve palsies (e.g. sudden onset of squint). If papilloedema, hypertension, bradycardia or focal signs are present an urgent CT or MRI brain scan is indicated. The majority of brain tumours are in the posterior fossa or brainstem, so the site of the pain is usually non-specific. They will often have cranial nerve palsies or cerebellar signs. See also Chapter 49.

Other causes of headache

Headaches are most often a feature of minor non-specific viral infections. These should be treated with simple analgesia such as paracetamol. Dental caries, sinusitis and otitis media are all treatable local infections that can cause headache. If headaches seem particularly related to school it is worth checking the child's visual acuity and recommend they see an optician. Always consider whether the headaches may be a manifestation of anxiety about school—is the child being bullied, or do the parents have unreasonable expectations?

KEY POINTS

- Headache is a common symptom in adolescence and is usually benign.
- Tension headaches are like a constricting band.
- Migraine often has visual symptoms and nausea, and there may be a family history.
- Parents are often worried about brain tumours. Raised intracranial pressure, focal neurological signs or unusual features are indications for brain imaging.

Types of fits, faints and funny turns

In infants and toddlers

Apnoea and acute life-threatening events (Chapter 67)
• Found limp or twitching
• Age: <6 months old
• Usually no precipitating event, but consider reflux, sepsis, arrhythmia

▶ **Febrile convulsions**
• Age: 6 months to 5 years
• Occurs on sudden rise of fever
• Lasts a few minutes

Breath holding spells (cyanotic)
• Older babies and toddlers
• Always precipitated by crying from pain or anger
• Stops breathing, becomes cyanotic and then limp
• No postictal state

Reflex anoxic spells (pallid)
• Precipitated by minor injury
• Turns pale and collapses
• Rapid recovery

▶ **Infantile spasms**
• A form of myoclonic epilepsy
• Jacknife spasms occurring in clusters
• Developmental regression

Hypoglycaemia and metabolic conditions
• Rare
• Always check blood sugar in any collapsed or unconscious child

In school-age children

Epilepsy (see Chapter 41)
Simple absence
• Fleeting vacant look
• 3 per second spike and wave on EEG

Partial epilepsy
• Twitching or jerking of face, arm or leg

Complex partial epilepsy
• Altered or impaired consciousness with strange sensations or semi-purposeful movements such as chewing or sucking
• May have postictal phase

Myoclonic epilepsy
• Shock-like jerks causing sudden falls
• Usually occurs in children with known neurological disability

Syncope (vasovagal)
• Precipitated by pain, emotion or prolonged standing
• Blurred vision, light-headedness, sweating, nausea
• Resolves on lying down

Hyperventilation
• Precipitated by excitement
• Excessive deep breathing, sometimes tetany
• Resolves on breathing into a paper bag

▶ **Cardiac arrhythmias**
• Palpitations may occur

What you need from your evaluation

History

• Obtain a description of the episode. Try to visualize the episode and 'replay' back to the witness. What was the child doing at the onset? Were there any precipitating factors? How long did it last? Was there loss or altered consciousness, involuntary movements, or a change in colour (pallor or cyanosis)? How did the child react to the event and was there a postictal phase?
• Home video recording—if episodes occur frequently, the parents may be able to obtain footage of an episode using a camcorder. This can provide excellent diagnostic information
• A developmental history is particularly important if infantile spasms or metabolic conditions are being considered
• Family history: is there anyone in the family with developmental problems, febrile seizures or a metabolic disorder? Is there a family history of cardiac arrhythmia (e.g. hypertrophic cardiomyopathy)? This is especially important if palpitations are a prominent feature of the history

Physical examination

• Rarely helpful between episodes
• Undertake a careful cardiac and neurological examination
• Dysmorphic features, micro- or macrocephaly and hepatosplenomegaly suggest a metabolic disorder

Investigations and their significance

The diagnosis is essentially clinical, but investigations must be considered if apnoea, epilepsy or a metabolic problem is suspected

• EEG — Hypsarrhythmia seen in infantile spasms
— 3 per second spike and wave activity in absence seizures
— Epileptiform activity may be seen in epilepsy (but may be present in normal children)

• ECG — Check cardiac rhythm, PR and QT intervals on 12-lead ECG

• 24 h ECG — If arrhythmia is suspected of causing syncope

• Blood chemistry — Hypoglycaemia, but unhelpful between episodes

• pH monitoring — Apnoea in infants may be due to GOR

Fits, faints and funny turns refer to episodes of transient altered consciousness, which usually present to the doctor after the event is over and may occur recurrently. They may cause great anxiety, although the child is often completely well in between episodes. A good description of the event should allow the different causes to be distinguished from each other, and it can be helpful to ask the family to video the episode. Most of the causes are benign and resolve with age. However, some forms of epilepsy can present in this way and need to be considered in the differential diagnosis. These include absence seizures, focal seizures such as temporal lobe seizures, and myoclonic seizures, which are covered in more detail in Chapter 41.

Breath-holding spells

Breath-holding spells (cyanotic spells) occur primarily in babies and toddlers. They normally resolve by 18 months of age. These spells are characteristically precipitated by crying due to pain or temper. The child cries once or twice, takes a deep breath, stops breathing, becomes deeply cyanotic and the limbs extend. Transient loss of consciousness may occur and even convulsive jerks. The child then becomes limp, resumes breathing and after a few seconds is fully alert again. The whole episode may last up to a minute. The key to diagnosis is the typical onset with crying and breath-holding and the absence of a postictal phase. The spells can sometimes occur several times a week and parents are often so terrified of them that they change their behaviour to avoid upsetting the child. They need to be reassured and encouraged to treat the child normally. There is no association with behavioural disorders.

Reflex anoxic seizures

These are also known as pallid spells or 'white' breath-holding attacks. The peak age is in toddlers from 6 months to 2 years. They classically follow a bump on the head or other minor injury, which triggers an excessive vagal reflex, causing transient bradycardia and circulatory impairment. The child may or may not cry, but then turns pale and collapses. There is transient apnoea and limpness followed by rapid recovery after 30–60 seconds. There may be eye-rolling and incontinence, and sometimes clonic stiffening of the limbs, but no tongue biting. After an attack the child may be tired and emotional for a few hours. The typical history and absence of postictal drowsiness helps distinguish these spells from epilepsy. Despite their appearance the attacks are always benign and disappear before school age. Parents need to be reassured and taught to put the child in the recovery position and await recovery.

Infantile spasms

Infantile spasms (West's syndrome) are a form of generalized myoclonic epilepsy (see Chapter 41) which can sometimes cause diagnostic confusion with other causes of loss of consciousness in young children. The onset is usually in infancy, peaking between 4–8 months. Characteristically there is a sudden tonic flexor spasm of the head and trunk causing the child to bend forwards ('salaam' attack). Relaxation occurs after a few seconds and the episode may reoccur in clusters up to 10 or 20 times. Clusters are commoner on awakening or just before sleep. Extensor spasms are sometimes seen. The EEG is diagnostic, showing a chaotic hypsarrhythmia pattern. In 20–30% there is an association with tuberous sclerosis,

so examination of the skin using a Wood's light is important. Infantile spasms are usually associated with severe learning disability. Treatment with vigabatrin may be beneficial.

Syncope (fainting)

Syncope occurs when there is hypotension and decreased cerebral perfusion. It occurs particularly in teenage girls reacting to painful or emotional stimuli, or prolonged standing. Blurring of vision, light-headedness, sweating and nausea precede loss of consciousness which is rapidly regained on lying flat. It is rarely a symptom of cardiac arrhythmias or poor cardiac output in childhood. Evaluation includes a cardiac examination, standing and lying blood pressure, and an ECG if there is doubt as to the cause of the faint. In unusually severe cases diagnosis may be helped by a tilt-table test, where the patient's ECG and blood pressure are measured while being tilted from lying to standing.

Cardiac arrhythmias

These are a rare cause of syncope, but should be considered if there is a clear history of preceding palpitations or if there is a family history of cardiac tachyarrhythmias or sudden death. Hypertrophic cardiomyopathy is an autosomal dominant condition that may present with syncope due to episodic ventricular tachycardia. Wolff–Parkinson–White syndrome causes supraventricular tachycardia due to re-entry rhythms and has a characteristic ECG with a short PR interval and a delta wave upstroke to the R wave. A markedly increased QT interval on the ECG may be associated with ventricular tachycardia and syncope. A 24-hour ECG recording may be useful in selected cases.

Hyperventilation

Excitement in some children, particularly teenage girls, may precipitate hyperventilation to the point of losing consciousness. The hyperventilation causes the carbon dioxide level to fall, triggering apnoea. The diagnosis is usually evident: breathing is excessive and deep, and tetany may also occur. Rebreathing into a paper bag allows the carbon dioxide level to rise and restores the child to normality. If episodes occur frequently, psychological therapy may be required.

Hypoglycaemia and other metabolic conditions

Metabolic disturbance, including hypoglycaemia, may cause loss of consciousness with seizures or a less dramatic alteration in consciousness. An underlying metabolic problem should be suspected if there are features such as developmental delay, dysmorphism, hepatosplenomegaly, or micro- or macrocephaly. Hypoglycaemia may be suspected if the episodes have a temporal relationship of to eating.

KEY POINTS

- Most fits, faints and funny turns are benign.
- A good history from a witness is crucial as the episodes are rarely observed by the doctor.
- The diagnosis is nearly always made on the basis of the history. Physical examination does not often contribute.
- Only carry out investigations if merited by the nature of the episode.

Generalized seizures

Generalized tonic–clonic epilepsy
- Tonic phase: sudden loss of consciousness, limbs extend, back arches, teeth clench, breathing stops tongue may be bitten
- Clonic phase: intermittent jerking movements irregular breathing may urinate and salivate
- Postictal phase: child sleepy and disorientated

Absence seizures
- Fleeting (5–20 seconds) impairment of consciousness (daydreaming)
- No falling or involuntary movements
- EEG: characteristic bursts of 3/second spike and wave activity

Infantile spasms (West's syndrome)
- A form of generalized myoclonic seizures
- Onset usually at 3-8 months of age
- Flexion spasms ('jacknife' or 'salaam')
- Last a few seconds, in clusters lasting up to half an hour
- Regression of developmental skills
- May have a history of perinatal asphyxia or meningitis
- EEG— characteristic hypsarrhythmic pattern
- Usually occur in children with a structural neurological degenerative condition

Focal seizures

Temporal lobe seizures
- Altered or impaired consciousness associated with strange sensations, hallucinations or semi-purposeful movements
- May show chewing, sucking or swallowing movements
- Postictal phase with amnesia
- EEG may show discharges arising from the temporal lobe

Seizure types according to the International League Against Epilepsy (ILAE) classification
- Generalized
- Generalized tonic–clonic seizures
- Tonic seizures
- Absence seizures
- Myoclonic seizures
- Atonic seizures
- Focal
- Focal motor seizures
- Focal sensory seizures
- Focal according to likely location
- Frontal lobe seizures
- Temporal lobe seizures
- Parietal lobe seizures
- Occipital lobe seizures

Prevalence
- Approximately 4 per 1000 schoolchildren

Pathophysiology
- Paroxysmal involuntary disturbances of brain function result in recurrent fits

How the diagnosis is made
- The diagnosis is largely clinical, based on the description of the attacks. EEG has a limited value in the diagnostic process
- Ask yourself four key questions:
  1. Is the seizure epilepsy?
  2. What sort of seizure is it?
  3. What sort of epilepsy is it?
  4. What is the cause of the epilepsy?

Prognosis
- Generally good, with resolution of fits in >70% of children with idiopathic epilepsy. Poor prognosis for those with infantile spasms

Paediatric follow-up
Monitor:
- Frequency of fits
- Side effects of drugs
- Psychosocial and educational problems
- Anticonvulsant levels if uncontrolled

Seizures, convulsions or *fits* are non-specific terms describing any impairment of consciousness, abnormal motor activity, sensory disturbance or autonomic dysfunction. *Epilepsy* is a specific diagnosis defined as a condition where fits are recurrent, resulting from paroxysmal involuntary disturbances of brain function that are unrelated to fever or acute cerebral insult. Seizures may be *generalized* from the onset, or *focal*, when they begin in a localized or focal area of the brain. Focal fits can be motor, sensory or autonomic, or a mixture of these three, and can become generalized. Epilepsy is usually idiopathic, but may result from a cerebral insult or underlying anatomical lesion, when it is called secondary. In some children, an insult or neurological problem is suspected but cannot be found and this type of epilepsy is cryptogenic.

The diagnosis of epilepsy is clinical, the key being a good detailed history. Physical examination is usually normal, but the finding of neurological signs suggests an underlying pathology. Investigations are not usually helpful as 50% of children with epilepsy have normal EEGs on first testing, and 5% of normal children have abnormal EEGs. EEG is useful in diagnosing certain syndromes, e.g. childhood absence epilepsy (previously called petit mal) and West's syndrome (infantile spasms). Twenty-four hour and video EEG recordings are sometimes helpful. MRI is usually indicated in children with focal epilepsy, and CT scans in acute neurological insults.

Medical management of epilepsy

The goal is to achieve the greatest control of fits while producing the least degree of side-effects. This is best achieved through a monotherapy approach:
- Treatment is started with the most effective drug for the type of fit.
- The dose is gradually increased to maximum recommended levels.
- A second drug is added if the first is ineffective, and the dose increased.
- The first drug, where possible, is gradually discontinued.
- Drugs should be given at intervals no longer than one half-life. Drugs with sedative effects should be given at bedtime and, if there is a pattern, the peak level should be timed to coincide with the seizures.

Most children are started on sodium valproate or carbamazepine, except for those with infantile spasms when steroid or vigabatrin (if associated with tuberous sclerosis) is the first line treatment. Ethosuxamide is an alternative to valproate for children with absence seizures only. If medical treatment fails, surgery may rarely be tried in children with intractable fits and clinical and electrographic evidence of a discrete epileptic focus. For most children with epilepsy restriction of physical activity is unnecessary, other than attendance by a responsible adult while bathing and swimming. As with any child, a helmet is recommended when cycling. Avoiding cycling in traffic and climbing high gymnastic equipment is prudent.

It is recommended that newly diagnosed children should receive support from an epilepsy nurse. The National Society for Epilepsy is a good source of information and support for the children and families.

Management of a tonic–clonic seizure

In a tonic–clonic seizure, the child should be placed in the recovery position after the fit is over. If the fit lasts for more than 10 minutes, parents should be instructed to end it by giving buccal midazolam or rectal diazepam. Intravenous drugs should only be given in hospital where facilities are available in the event of respiratory arrest. Children do not need to be hospitalized each time a fit occurs. Emergency treatment is not required for other forms of epileptic fits.

Monitoring a child with epilepsy

The family should be encouraged to keep a diary recording any fits along with medications received, side-effects and behavioural changes. This allows you to accurately review the child's condition and the effect of drugs. Physical examination is not required at every visit but should be carried out if there is a deterioration in control. Monitoring of anticonvulsant blood levels is not routine but is helpful if fits are uncontrolled or drug toxicity is suspected. Levels below the therapeutic range can result from inadequate dosage, poor absorption, rapid drug metabolism, drug interactions and deliberate or accidental non-compliance.

Living with epilepsy

Epilepsy is a difficult condition for children to live with as it periodically and unpredictably places them in embarrassing situations. They may suffer from stigmatization and social difficulties, and their integration into school may become affected. Too often physical activities are limited for fear that a fit will place the child in danger.

Most parents are initially frightened by the diagnosis of epilepsy and require support and accurate information about the condition. They need to know how to safely manage an acute fit including using buccal midazolam or rectal diazepam, about side effects of drugs, the dangers of sudden withdrawal of medication, and social and academic repercussions. There may be concern about genetic implications, and it is important that teenage girls know about the teratogenic effects of anticonvulsants.

Families may need to be encouraged to treat their child as normally as possible and not to thwart their independence. This often becomes a particular issue in adolescence when compliance too can be a problem. Career guidance is important as some occupations are closed to individuals with epilepsy. Application for a driving licence can only be made after one fit-free year whether the person is on or off medication.

Staff at school must be taught the correct management of tonic–clonic seizures. Teachers need to be aware of other types of fit such as absence seizures, as well as side-effects of drugs, and report these to the parents or school nurse. When epilepsy is associated with learning difficulties, appropriate help needs to be provided.

KEY POINTS

- Ensure the diagnosis is correct.
- Only treat if fits are recurrent.
- Use monotherapy when possible.
- Check plasma levels if control is inadequate and, if low, consider non-compliance.
- For tonic–clonic epilepsy, buccal midazolam or rectal diazepam should be prescribed for home use.
- Ensure any learning difficulties are addressed.
- Help the child live a normal life with full participation at school and home.

Cerebral palsy is a disorder of movement caused by a permanent, non-progressive lesion in the developing brain. Spastic cerebral palsy is the most common form where the injury is in the cerebral cortex or motor pathways. Athetoid and ataxic cerebral palsy are less common

Hemiplegia
- One side of the body
- Arm often more involved than the leg
- Delayed walking
- Tiptoe gait, with arm in a dystonic posture when running

Diplegia
- Both legs involved with arms less affected or unaffected
- Excessive hip adduction (hard to put on a nappy)
- Scissoring of legs
- Characteristic gait: feet in equinovarus and walking on tiptoe

Athetoid cerebral palsy
- Due to basal ganglia damage
- Writhing movements
- Intelligence often normal
- Major physical impairment

Total body impairment
- Most severe form
- All extremities involved
- High association with severe learning disabilities and fits
- Swallowing difficulties and gastro-oesophageal reflux common
- Flexion contractures of the knees and elbows often present by late childhood

Ataxic cerebral palsy
- Due to cerebral damage
- Poor coordination
- Ataxic gait

Prevalence
- 2 per 1000 children

Aetiology
- Prenatal   Cerebral malformations
  Congenital infection
  Metabolic defects

- Perinatal   Complications of prematurity
  Intrapartum trauma
  Hypoxic–ischaemic insult

- Postnatal   Non-accidental injury
  (injury incurred   Head trauma
  before 2 years   Meningitis/encephalitis
  of age)   Cardiopulmonary arrest

Diagnosis

Diagnosis is clinical, based on the findings of abnormalities of tone, delays in motor development, abnormal movement patterns and persistent primitive reflexes. Diagnosis may be suspected in neonates but can only be made months later

Associated problems

Children with cerebral palsy may commonly have additional problems (especially if they are quadriplegic or severe hemiplegic):
- Learning difficulties
- Epilepsy
- Visual impairment
- Squint
- Hearing loss
- Speech disorders
- Behaviour disorders
- Undernutrition and poor growth
- Respiratory problems

Prognosis

Depends on the degree and type of cerebral palsy, level of learning diasability and presence of other associated problems. The degree of independent living achieved relates to:
- Type and extent of cerebral palsy
- Degree of learning disability
- Presence of associated problems, e.g. visual impairment, epilepsy

Cerebral palsy is a disorder of movement and posture caused by a permanent and non-progressive cerebral lesion acquired early in brain development. It is often complicated by other neurological and learning difficulties. Although the brain lesion itself in cerebral palsy is non-progressive, the clinical picture changes as the child grows and develops. The underlying brain lesion may result from different insults occurring at various times in the developing brain.

In the neonatal period cerebral palsy may be suspected if a baby has difficulty sucking, irritability, convulsions, or an abnormal neurological examination. The diagnosis is usually made later in the first year when the following features emerge.

• **Abnormalities of tone:** Initially the tone may be reduced, but eventually spasticity develops.
• **Delay in motor development:** Such as marked head lag, delays in sitting and rolling over.
• **Abnormal patterns of development:** Movements are not only delayed, but also abnormal in quality.
• **Persistence of primitive reflexes:** Such as the Moro, grasp and asymmetric tonic neck reflex.

The diagnosis is made on clinical grounds, with repeated examinations often required to establish the diagnosis. Once made, a multidisciplinary assessment is needed to define the extent of the difficulties. An MRI scan is useful to demonstrate cerebral injury or malformations, delineating their extent and ruling out very rare progressive or treatable causes such as tumours.

Management of cerebral palsy

Most children with cerebral palsy have multiple difficulties and require a multidisciplinary input. This is provided by a Child Development Team, involving a paediatrician, physiotherapist, occupational therapist, speech and language therapist, health visitor and psychologist. They structure a coordinated programme of treatment to meet all the child's needs, and ensure good liaison between professionals and parents.

Therapy
Physiotherapy

Physiotherapists advise on handling and mobilization, and their role is crucial. The family must be taught how to handle the child in daily activities such as feeding, carrying, dressing and bathing in ways that limit the effects of abnormal muscle tone. They are also taught a series of exercises to prevent the development of deforming contractures. The physiotherapist may also provide a variety of aids, such as firm boots, lightweight splints and walking frames for the child when beginning to walk.

Occupational therapy

The role of the occupational therapist overlaps with that of the physiotherapist. The occupational therapist is trained to advise on equipment such as wheelchairs and seating, and on play materials and activities that best encourage the child's hand function.

Speech therapy

The speech and language therapist is involved on two accounts— feeding and language. In the early months advice may be required for feeding and swallowing difficulties. Later, a thorough assessment of the child's developing speech and language is required and help given on all aspects of communication, including non-verbal systems when necessary.

Paediatric management

The paediatrician's key role is supportive, and involves liaison with other professionals, including school. In the long term the child needs to be monitored for developmental progress, medical problems, including epilepsy, development of contractures or joint dislocation, behavioural difficulties and nutritional status. Drugs, other than anticonvulsants for epilepsy, have a limited role in cerebral palsy. However, newer therapies include intramuscular botulinum toxin to relax hypertonic muscle groups and intrathecal baclofen via subcutaneous pump infusion for spasticity.

Orthopaedic problems

Even with adequate physiotherapy, orthopaedic deformities may develop as a result of long-standing muscle weakness or spasticity. Dislocation of the hip may occur as a result of spasticity in the thigh adductors and preschool children at risk require routine hip radiographs to ensure this is identified. Fixed equinus deformity of the ankle may develop as a result of calf muscle spasticity.

Nutrition

Undernutrition commonly occurs in children with cerebral palsy, and can reduce the child's chances of achieving their physical and intellectual potential. Food must be given in a form appropriate to the child's ability to chew and swallow. Energy-rich supplements and medical treatment for reflux may be required. A child who is unable to eat adequate amounts may need a gastrostomy to meet nutritional needs. Over time some children lose the ability to swallow safely, placing them at risk for aspiration. In this circumstance oral feeds must be discontinued.

Growing up with cerebral palsy

The family has to cope with all the difficulties facing any family with a disabled child. However, cerebral palsy, if severe, places particularly heavy demands in terms of time and input. Everyday tasks such as dressing and bathing take time, and feeding, in particular, may take hours each day. The child also needs regular physiotherapy at home, and needs to attend appointments, both for medical follow-up and therapy. In view of this the family needs support, often beyond what family and friends can supply. Voluntary and social service agencies can provide babysitting, respite care and financial support.

Children with milder forms of cerebral palsy can cope at mainstream school, provided minor learning difficulties and physical access are addressed. Children with more severe cerebral palsy may need special schooling in a school for the physically or severely learning disabled, depending on the degree of their difficulties.

KEY POINTS

• Physiotherapy is needed to minimize the effects of spasticity and prevent contractures.
• Associated problems must be identified and managed.
• Any special educational needs must be met.
• The family needs adequate financial, practical and emotional support.
• The child's integration into society should be maximized.

Joint inflammation

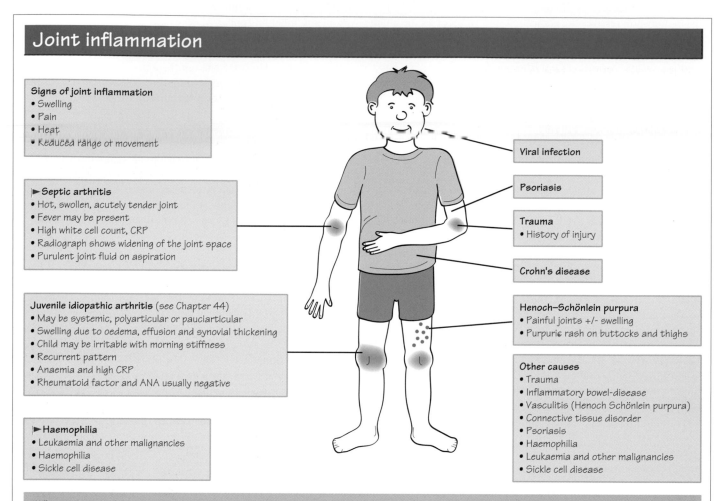

Signs of joint inflammation
- Swelling
- Pain
- Heat
- Reduced range of movement

►Septic arthritis
- Hot, swollen, acutely tender joint
- Fever may be present
- High white cell count, CRP
- Radiograph shows widening of the joint space
- Purulent joint fluid on aspiration

Juvenile idiopathic arthritis (see Chapter 44)
- May be systemic, polyarticular or pauciarticular
- Swelling due to oedema, effusion and synovial thickening
- Child may be irritable with morning stiffness
- Recurrent pattern
- Anaemia and high CRP
- Rheumatoid factor and ANA usually negative

►Haemophilia
- Leukaemia and other malignancies
- Haemophilia
- Sickle cell disease

Viral infection

Psoriasis

Trauma
- History of injury

Crohn's disease

Henoch–Schönlein purpura
- Painful joints +/- swelling
- Purpuric rash on buttocks and thighs

Other causes
- Trauma
- Inflammatory bowel-disease
- Vasculitis (Henoch Schönlein purpura)
- Connective tissue disorder
- Psoriasis
- Haemophilia
- Leukaemia and other malignancies
- Sickle cell disease

What you need from your evaluation

History
- **Joint symptoms:** in most conditions pain is exacerbated by activity but in inflammatory arthropathies joint stiffness is alleviated by exercise
- Are there **systemic symptoms?** Fever, anorexia, weight loss, rash, weakness and fatigue suggest systemic causes
- **Past medical and family history:** important information includes previous arthritis, inflammatory bowel disease, autoimmune conditions, blood dyscrasias and psoriasis

Investigations and their significance

Full blood count	Signs of bacterial infection, anaemia in chronic disease, haemoglobinopathies, malignancy
CRP and plasma viscosity	Elevated in bacterial infection, collagen vascular disease and inflammatory bowel disease
Blood culture	Positive in septic arthritis
ASOT	High in reactive arthritis or, very rarely, rheumatic fever
Viral titres	Viral arthritis
Rheumatoid factor and antinuclear antibodies	Negative in most forms of juvenile chronic arthritis
Radiography of the joint	Characteristics differ with underlying aetiology
Joint aspiration	Microscopy and culture to exclude or confirm septic arthritis
MRI of joint	Can identify soft tissue injury (muscle, cartilage) and may show oedema and effusions

Physical examination
- **Musculoskeletal system:** examine all four limbs and the spine. Look for skin colour changes, heat, tenderness, range of motion and asymmetry
- **Observe** the child's gait
- **General examination:** look for anaemia, hepatosplenomegaly, cardiac murmurs and rash
- **Check for focus of infection:** Staphylococcus aureus can cause widespread septic emboli including septic arthritis or osteomyelitis
- **Check adjoining joints:** a painful knee may be due to problems at the hip or ankle

Key points
- Causes other than traumatic are rare
- If the joint is acutely swollen, rule out septic arthritis as the cause
- Always enquire about systemic symptoms
- Clues to the underlying diagnosis are provided by the history and distribution of the joints involved

Paediatrics at a Glance, Third Edition. Lawrence Miall, Mary Rudolf, Dominic Smith. © 2012 John Wiley & Sons, Ltd. Published 2012 by John Wiley & Sons, Ltd.

Juvenile idiopathic arthritis

Juvenile idiopathic arthritis (JIA) is a group of conditions that present in childhood with joint inflammation lasting 6 weeks for which no other cause is found. Up to 1 in 1000 children may be affected during childhood. The classification depends on the presentation, but may not be reliably assigned for 6 months. Treatment is aimed at treating the pain and inflammation and maintaining good joint mobility. In the majority there is resolution during childhood. A multidisciplinary approach with psychological support is necessary for these children

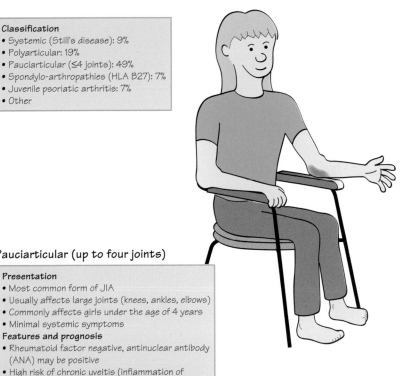

Classification
- Systemic (Still's disease): 9%
- Polyarticular: 19%
- Pauciarticular (≤4 joints): 49%
- Spondylo-arthropathies (HLA B27): 7%
- Juvenile psoriatic arthritis: 7%
- Other

Pauciarticular (up to four joints)

Presentation
- Most common form of JIA
- Usually affects large joints (knees, ankles, elbows)
- Commonly affects girls under the age of 4 years
- Minimal systemic symptoms

Features and prognosis
- Rheumatoid factor negative, antinuclear antibody (ANA) may be positive
- High risk of chronic uveitis (inflammation of anterior eye structures), especially if ANA +ve. Needs regular slit-lamp examination to screen for this
- Arthritis resolves completely in 80%

Systemic onset (Still's disease)

Presentation
- Spiking fever, severe malaise
- Salmon-pink rash
- Anaemia, weight loss
- Hepatosplenomegaly, pericarditis
- Arthralgia and myalgia but may have minimal joint symptoms
- May resemble malignancy

Features
- Both large and small joints affected
- 25% have severe arthritis
- Rheumatoid factor negative
- Temporomandibular joint may be involved, causing micrognathia
- Associated with HLA-DR4

Prognosis
- In 25%, arthritis persists into adulthood with disability
- May require joint replacements

Polyarticular (more than 4 joints)

Presentation
- Symmetrical involvement of large and small joints
- There may be poor weight gain and mild anaemia
- Morning stiffness
- Irritability in young children

Features and prognosis
- Rheumatoid factor negative in 97%, ANA may be positive
- No eye involvement
- 12% develop severe arthritis but prognosis is generally good

Management

The aims of management are to preserve joint function, to minimize complications, including complications of the treatment, and to aid the psychological adjustment to what can be a chronic disabling condition in some.

The aim is to reduce joint inflammation using non-steroidal anti-inflammatory drugs (NSAIDs). Steroids may be injected into affected joints. Disease modifying drugs are used if steroid injections need to be repeated frequently. These include methotrexate and immunosuppressants such as ciclosporin, azathioprine and systemic steroids. All have side effects. A new class of recombinant antibody drugs has been introduced which act as biological agents to reduce TNF action. These drugs are used when methotrexate is not fully controlling the inflammation (includes etanercept, infliximab, adalimumab). Non-drug therapy includes physiotherapy, hydrotherapy and wearing splints to maintain joint function and mobility. Occupational therapy can help with aids to improve function. The family needs psychological support. Children with residual disability may require help in planning a suitable career

Investigations

ESR	Raised in systemic form, may be raised in polyarticular but normal in pauciarticular arthritis
FBC	Microcytic anaemia of chronic disease
Autoantibody	(ANA) +ve in 25% (especially pauciarticluar)
Rheumatoid factor	Rarely positive – marker for persistence of polyarticular arthritis into adulthood
Radiology	Radiography and MRI of affected joints
Echo	In systemic form to exclude pericarditis

Complications

Flexion contractures of the joint may develop without regular therapy and splinting. Joint destruction may require eventual joint replacement (e.g. knees, hips) in some children. Growth failure can occur due to the chronic illness, anorexia and the growth suppression effect of corticosteroid therapy. Chronic anterior uveitis (iridocyclitis) is asymptomatic but if missed can lead to visual impairment.

Causes of leg pain and limp in childhood

Growing pains
- Preschool children
- Pain often at night, but no limp by day
- Often bilateral and felt in shins or thighs
- Pain predominantly in muscles not bone
- Healthy child, no physical signs
- No interference with normal activities

Transient synovitis
- Benign and common in boys aged 2–8 years
- Sudden onset of limp
- No systemic symptoms
- Often preceded by URTI
- Normal investigations and radiographs

Septic arthritis (see Chapter 43)
- Infant and toddler
- Looks septic
- Swollen hot joint (not obvious in the hip)
- Serious condition

Trauma

Osteomyelitis
- Fever
- Swelling, erythema, tenderness, decreased movement of the limb
- High CRP, WCC
- Diagnosis by radiography, bone scan or MRI

Legg–Perthes disease
- Osteochondritis leading to avascular necrosis of femoral head
- 4:1 male to female ratio
- Age 4–11, peak 4–7 years
- May follow transient synovitis
- Initially painless
- Pain and limp when fracture occurs
- Diagnosis by radiography or MRI

Slipped capital femoral epiphysis
- Overweight teenage boys
- Gradual onset of pain in groin or knee
- Diagnosis by radiography

► Neoplastic disease
- Benign or malignant
- Pain, tenderness and mass
- Destructive mass on radiography
- Gnawing pain in leukaemia

What you need from your evaluation

History
- Organic pain tends to be persistent, occurring day and night, interrupts play as well as schooling, is often unilateral or located to a joint in particular
- A limp or refusal to walk is significant
- Weight loss, fever, night sweats, rash or diarrhoea point to organic causes

Physical examination
- Examine the child lying down and walking, and fully examine the leg and groin, not only the knee
- **The limb.** Look for point tenderness, redness, swelling, muscle weakness or atrophy, and limitation of movement for each joint
- **General examination.** Look for fever, rash, pallor, lymphadenopathy or organomegaly suggesting infectious or systemic causes

Investigations and their significance

(Only if leg pain is thought to be organic)

Full blood count	High white cell count in leukaemia, infections, collagen vascular disease
CRP, ESR or plasma viscosity	High in infections, collagen vascular disease, Inflammatory bowel disease, tumours
Radiography	Bone tumours, infection, trauma, avascular necrosis, leukaemia, slipped capital femoral epiphysis
MRI or bone scan	Osteomyelitis

Key points
- Organic and non-organic causes can be differentiated on clinical grounds. Leg pain alone is usually non-organic
- Important features suggestive of organic disease are a child's refusal to walk, a limp, any physical signs, or constitutional symptoms
- Pain in the hip is referred to the knee, so children presenting with knee pain require a full examination of the leg and groin

Common childhood skeletal problems

Skull
- Craniosynostosis
  - Premature fusion of skull sutures
  - Distorted head growth
  - Ridging of the sutures
  - Surgical correction needed if multiple sutures
- Plagiocephaply
  - Common asymmetry of the skull
  - Normal head circumference
  - Usually improves over the first few years

Plagiocephaply

Chest
- Outbowing (pectus carinatum)
- Incurving (pectus excavatum)
- Usually seen around adolescence
- Cosmetic effect can cause distress
- Surgical correction is an option

Arms and hands
- Absent (or extra) fingers seen
- Absence of a larger segment can occur
- Can be linked to other malformations (e.g VACTERL sequence)

Legs
- Bowlegged (genu varum)
- Knock-kneed (genu valgum)
  - Both common in preschool children
  - Usually resolve
  - Extreme bow-legged in rickets (vitamin D deficiency)

Genu varum   Genu valgum   Normal

18/12 months   3 yrs   6 yrs

Spine
- Spina bifida congenital defect
  - Neurological impairment, movement and continence problems
  - Linked with hydrocephalus
- Scoliosis
  - Growing adolescents
  - Children with neuromuscular disorders
  - Splinting or surgery may be needed

Scoliosis

Hip
- Congenital dysplasia of hip (CDH)
  - Increased risk with female sex, breech, family history
  - Screening examination (Barlow Ortolani exam)
  - Repeat surveillance until walking
- Perthes
  - Ischaemia at the growing femoral head
  - Pain, limping in young child
- Slipped upper femoral epiphysis
  - Hip pain and gait problems in older children and adolescents

Feet
- Talipes equinovarus
  - Common in newborns as a transient postural deformity
  - Rarely a more fixed deformity
  - Needs physiotherapy and surgery if persistent

Toe-walking
- Commonly a behavioural habit
- Usually normal legs
- Can be a sign of diplegic cerebral palsy

Flat feet (pes planus)
- Common in toddlers and does not impair walking
- In older children can cause knee pain
- Podiatry to correct with supportive instep

Causes of anaemia and pallor

Hypochromic microcytic anaemias

Iron deficiency anaemia
- Often asymptomatic
- Common in rapidly growing children
- Linked with poor diet, excessive cow's milk
- Low ferritin level proportional to stored iron

Thalassaemia trait
- Often asymptomatic
- Normal ferritin
- High HbA2, HbF = beta trait
- Low/Normal HbA2, HbF = alpha trait

Normochromic normocytic anaemia
- Chronic renal disease
- Hypothyroidism
- Chronic inflammatory disease
- Chronic infection

Lead poisoning
- Rare
- Pica (eating lead-containing material)
- Irritability, colic, encephalopathy

Haemolytic anaemia
- Hereditary spherocytosis
- Autoimmune haemolysis
- Red cell enzyme disorders (e.g. G6PD deficiency)
- Haemoglobinopathies (e.g. sickle cell)

Blood film showing hypochromic microcytic picture, poikilocytes and red cell fragments, typical of iron deficiency anaemia

Film showing abnormal blast cells in acute lymphoblastic leukaemia (© HMDS, Leeds)

Sickle cell disease (© microscopyU.com)

Other causes
- Chronic infection
- Chronic renal failure
- Malignancies

Other anaemias

Leukaemia (see Chapter 49)
- Insidious anorexia, irritability and lethargy
- Pallor
- Bleeding
- Fever
- Low Hb and platelets
- High white cell count with blast cells

Anaemia of marrow infiltration
- Leukaemia
- Lymphoma
- Histiocytosis
- Neuroblastoma
- Metabolic storage disorders

Bone marrow failure
- Leukaemia
- Aplastic anaemia
  e.g. congenital Fanconi anaemia
  acquired aplastic anaemia
  post infection

Sickle cell anaemia
- Affects black individuals
- Identified by Hb electrophoresis

What you need from your evaluation

History

- What is the child's diet like?
  Ask about consumption of milk. Early introduction of 'doorstep milk' causes microscopic bleeding from the gut. Excessive milk intake (>1 pint/day) after 12 months of age can reduce solid, and therefore iron, intake. Prolonged exclusive breast-feeding may lead to iron deficiency. Is the diet varied? Many young children are faddy about eating iron-rich foods. Ask about pica, which may be associated with lead ingestion
- Is there any history of bleeding e.g. menorrhagia in girls?
- What is the child's ethnic origin and is there consanguinity? Relevant for haemoglobinopathies
- What are the home conditions like?
  Could there be exposure to fumes or old lead paint?

Physical examination

- Carry out a full physical examination
- Anaemia has to be significant to be clinically apparent. It is best seen in the conjunctivae and nail beds
- Look for evidence of hepatosplenomegaly. This suggests more severe causes of anaemia

Investigations and their significance

- Full blood count — Severity and type of anaemia (microcytic, hypochromic, etc) Presence of bizarre cells. Presence of blast cells
- Ferritin — Low in iron deficiency
- Zn-protoporphyrin — Raised in iron deficiency and in lead poisoning
- Lead level — High in lead toxicity
- Haemoglobin electrophoresis — Abnormal in haemoglobinopathies
- Urea and electrolytes — Abnormal in renal failure
- Blood and urine culture — Chronic infection
- Bone marrow aspirate — Only needed if blast cells seen on peripheral film

Iron deficiency anaemia

In early childhood the combination of a high demand for iron to keep up with rapid growth and a poor intake of iron-rich foods makes iron deficiency very common. This can be exacerbated by chronic blood loss induced by early exposure to whole cow's milk. Iron deficiency anaemia can be as high as 50% in some populations, and in many countries young children are screened routinely. Babies beyond 12 months should be limited to 1 pint of milk (500 mL) daily to reduce blood loss and encourage the consumption of more iron-rich foods. Breast milk is somewhat protective as, although it has a relatively low iron content, the iron is absorbed more efficiently due to the iron binding protein, lactoferrin. However, exclusive breast-feeding beyond 6 months with delayed weaning can cause iron deficiency.

Iron deficiency anaemia is usually asymptomatic, but if the haemoglobin level falls significantly irritability and anorexia occur. Iron deficiency, even without anaemia, can affect attention span, alertness and learning. The initial finding is a low ferritin level reflecting inadequate iron stores. As the deficiency progresses microcytosis, hypochromia and poikilocytosis develop. Zn-protoporphyrin is high, as haem binds to zinc in the absence of iron. Treatment of iron deficiency is iron salts given orally for 2–3 months. The haemoglobin level starts to rise within 1 week of treatment. Failure to do so suggests non-compliance or an incorrect diagnosis. Patients should be warned that iron supplements make the stool turn black and that iron is dangerous in overdose. The medicines must be stored safely, away from toddlers.

Thalassaemia

The thalassaemias are a group of heritable hypochromic anaemias varying in severity, caused by a defect in haemoglobin polypeptide synthesis. Beta-thalassaemia is the commonest, and affects Asian and Mediterranean individuals (1 in 7 Cypriots, 1 in 20 Indians). Overall, 3% of the world's population carry the thalassaemia gene mutation.

Beta-thalassaemia trait (the heterozygous form) causes a mild hypochromic, microcytic anaemia, which may be confused with iron deficiency. Diagnosis is made by haemoglobin electrophoresis which demonstrates high levels of HbA2 and HbF. It requires no treatment. Alpha-thalassaemia trait (heterozygous) is suggested by a mild hypochromic microcytic anaemia with low or normal levels of HbA2 and HbF and no evidence of iron deficiency. It is important to recognize these conditions to avoid unnecessary iron treatment and to give patients advice that their own future children could be at risk of a more serious thalassaemia major disorder, so a future partner may need a thalassaemia screen.

Homozygous beta-thalassaemia results in a severe haemolytic anaemia, with compensatory bone marrow hyperplasia producing a characteristic bossing of the facial and skull bones and leads to dental abnormalities. There is marked hepatosplenomegaly. Blood transfusions are required on a regular basis to maintain haemoglobin levels. Haemosiderosis due to iron overload is an inevitable consequence causing cardiomyopathy, diabetes and skin pigmentation, but can be minimized by continuous subcutaneous infusions of the chelating agent desferrioxamine (deferoxamine).

Sickle-cell anaemia

Sickle-cell anaemia is the commonest haemoglobinopathy, occurring in 1 in 4 West Africans and 1 in 10 Afro-Caribbean people. In sickle cell disease one of the amino acid sequences in the beta-globin chain is substituted, causing an unstable haemoglobin (HbS). When deoxygenated, this forms highly structured polymers making brittle spiny red cells which occlude blood vessels, causing ischaemia. Heterozygote carriers (sickle cell trait) are usually asymptomatic, but can experience problems during general anaesthesia. There are over 300 haemoglobinopathies and other forms of sickle cell disease include HbSC or Hb-beta-Thal, where the child is a compound heterozygote, inheriting HbS from one parent and HbC or beta-thalassaemia trait from the other.

In the homozygous condition children experience recurrent acute painful crises which can be precipitated by dehydration, hypoxia, infection or acidosis. Painful swelling of the hands and feet is a common early presentation. Repeated splenic infarctions eventually leave the child asplenic and therefore susceptible to serious infections. Pneumococcal vaccination and prophylactic penicillin is recommended. Renal damage leads to a reduced ability to concentrate urine, making dehydration a severe problem. Treatment of a crisis is largely symptomatic with analgesics, antibiotics, warmth and adequate fluid hydration.

The peripheral blood film typically shows target cells, poikilocytes and irreversibly sickled cells. Diagnosis is made by haemoglobin electrophoresis, which may also be used for screening in susceptible populations. Universal antenatal screening is now offered to mothers and the newborn blood spot is screened for abnormal haemoglobin.

> ## KEY POINTS
>
> • Iron deficiency is common in children as it is hard to sustain iron stores in the face of rapid growth and a toddler's often low intake of iron-rich foods.
> • Iron deficiency anaemia usually responds to a 2-month therapeutic trial of iron. Further investigations are only needed if there is no response.
> • Principal causes of microcytic hypochromic anaemia include iron deficiency, lead poisoning and thalassemia trait.
> • If a child is ill or from an at-risk population then consider other causes of anaemia such as sickle cell disease.
> • Haemoglobinopathies can be detected in a newborn blood spot screening test.

Causes of jaundice in the neonatal period

Unconjugated hyperbilirubinaemia

Prematurity
- Immature liver enzymes

Rhesus incompatibility
- If mother is Rh negative and baby Rh positive, then maternal IgG can cause haemolysis
- Sensitization occurs in earlier pregnancies
- If severe can cause hydrops in utero
- Coombs' test positive

ABO incompatibility
- Usually milder than rhesus

Infection
- Bacterial infection

Bruising
- Skin or scalp bruising from traumatic delivery is broken down into bilirubin

Hypothyroidism
- May be associated with pituitary disease

▶ Breast milk jaundice
- Well baby who is breast-fed
- Jaundice develops in second week

▶ Physiological
- Low liver enzyme activity
- Breakdown of fetal haemoglobin

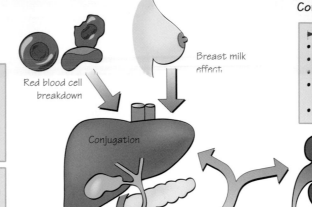

Red blood cell breakdown

Breast milk effect

Conjugation

Urobilinogen

Enterohepatic circulation

Stercobilinogen

Conjugated hyperbilirubinaemia

▶ Hepatitis
- Neonatal hepatitis
- Hepatitis A,B,C
- Congenital viral infection (e.g. CMV)
- Inborn errors of metabolism (e.g. galactosaemia)
- Abnormal liver function tests

Cystic fibrosis
- Cholestasis

Choledocal cyst

▶ Biliary atresia
- Persistent jaundice with rising conjugated fraction
- Pale, chalky stools
- Requires urgent referral for assessment, diagnostic isotope scan and surgical correction

What you need from your evaluation

History
- At what age did the jaundice develop? (within 24 h of birth always requires investigation)
- Are there any risk factors for infection?
- Is there a family history (cystic fibrosis, spherocytosis)?
- Is the baby active, alert and feeding well or lethargic and having to be woken for feeds (significant jaundice)

Examination
- What is the extent of the jaundice? (it tends to spread from the head down as it becomes more significant)
- Are there other features of congenital viral infection, such as petechiae, anaemia or hepatosplenomegaly?
- Is the baby dehydrated? Failure to establish breast-feeding may present with severe jaundice and hypernatraemia in the first week of life
- Is the baby well or are there signs of infection?
- Examine the stool—pale stools may indicate obstructive jaundice

Management
- Identify the cause and severity of the jaundice
- Use phototherapy to bring down the bilirubin level
- In severe haemolytic disease, multiple exchange transfusions may be required to prevent kernicterus
- Management of conjugated jaundice depends on cause but refer early to hepatologist if biliary atresia is suspected
- Prolonged jaundice can increase the chance of bleeding disorders associated with vitamin K deficiency. Check coagulation screen and give further vitamin K supplements

Investigations and their significance

• Split bilirubin	Total bilirubin and conjugated fraction (should be <20%)
• FBC	Thrombocytopenia suggests viral infection or IUGR
	Anaemia in haemolytic disease
	Neutropenia or neutrophilia in infection
• Group and Coombs'	ABO and rhesus incompatibility
• Thyroid function	Hypothyroidism
• TORCH screen	Hepatitis B, cytomegalovirus infection
• LFTs	A high alanine transaminase (ALT) suggests hepatitis
• Urine metabolic screen	Inborn errors of metabolism
• Liver ultrasound	To visualize biliary tree
• Infection screen	Urine, blood and cerebrospinal fluid
• Liver isotope scan	To rule out biliary atresia in persistent conjugated hyperbilirubinaemia
• Coagulation	Clotting factors are not synthesized well in liver disease, and obstructive jaundice may cause vitamin K deficiency

Jaundice is the yellow pigmentation of the skin that occurs with hyperbilirubinaemia. The bilirubin is formed from the breakdown of haem in red blood cells and is transported to the liver as unconjugated bilirubin, bound to albumin. In order to be excreted it needs to be made water soluble by conjugation in the liver. Conjugated bilirubin is then excreted in the bile into the duodenum, where some is reabsorbed (the enterohepatic circulation) and the remainder forms stercobilinogen, which gives the stools their yellow/brown pigment. Some of the reabsorbed conjugated bilirubin is excreted by the kidneys as urobilinogen.

Excessive haemolysis or impaired conjugation leads to a build-up of unconjugated bilirubin, and obstruction to drainage of bile leads to conjugated hyperbilirubinaemia. Unconjugated and unbound bilirubin is lipid soluble and can cross the blood–brain barrier.

Kernicterus

If free bilirubin crosses the blood–brain barrier in high concentrations it is deposited in the basal ganglia where it causes *kernicterus*. This causes an acute encephalopathy with irritability, high-pitched cry or coma. The neurotoxic damage to the basal ganglia can lead to the development of athetoid cerebral palsy. Kernicterus is now extremely rare due to better obstetric management of rhesus disease, careful monitoring of bilirubin levels and early treatment with phototherapy. Extremely sick preterm infants are still at risk of kernicterus, especially if they are acidotic or have a low serum albumin.

Treatment

Phototherapy (blue light at 450nm wavelength) helps convert unconjugated bilirubin to biliverdin, an isomer which can be excreted by the kidneys. In rhesus or ABO incompatibility, if bilirubin levels rise significantly despite phototherapy, then an exchange transfusion is required to remove the bilirubin and the maternal IgG antibodies from the circulation. Intravenous immunoglobulin infusion can help prevent the need for exchange transfusion by blocking antibody receptor sites.

Physiological jaundice

Jaundice in the neonatal period is very common and is usually due to liver immaturity. It is self-limiting as liver enzymes mature over the first week, and only occasionally needs phototherapy treatment. Nearly all preterm infants become jaundiced in the first days of life, due to the immature hepatocytes not being able to adequately conjugate bilirubin. This never requires exchange transfusion but may require phototherapy for a few days.

Breast-milk jaundice

Persistent jaundice in an otherwise well breast-fed infant with normal-coloured stools and urine is probably due to the inhibition of liver conjugation enzymes by substances in breast milk. It is a diagnosis of exclusion and a split bilirubin should be measured to exclude conjugated hyperbilirubinaemia. Breast-milk jaundice normally manifests itself by day 4–7 and can persist for 3 weeks to 3 months. Breast-milk jaundice should be distinguished from the severe jaundice and hypernatraemic dehydration that can occasionally occur in the first week of life due to failure to establish adequate lactation.

Haemolytic disease of the newborn

Haemolysis occurs when maternal IgG antibody crosses the placenta and reacts with fetal red blood cell antigens. The commonest causes are ABO or rhesus incompatibility. In rhesus disease the fetus is rhesus positive and the mother rhesus negative. The mother will have been sensitized by the passage of fetal red blood cells into her circulation at a previous delivery or during a threatened miscarriage. Rhesus-negative women are now routinely immunized with anti-D antibody at 28 weeks, to 'mop up' fetal red blood cells before they stimulate maternal IgG production. Fetal anaemia can lead to hydrops (severe oedema). In-utero blood transfusions can now be given (via the umbilical cord) in severe cases of haemolytic disease. After birth untreated fetuses are anaemic and rapidly develop severe jaundice. The management of severe disease is to deliver the baby before severe haemolysis has occurred and then to wash out the maternal antibodies (and the bilirubin) by performing a series of exchange transfusions, and by the aggressive use of early phototherapy. It is important to remember that the maternal IgG antibodies can persist in the baby's circulation for many weeks, causing ongoing haemolysis and anaemia even after the jaundice is under control.

Biliary atresia

Biliary atresia is a rare (1 in 10000) but important condition caused by the absence of intra- or extrahepatic bile ducts. A conjugated hyperbilirubinaemia develops over weeks, and the stools become clay coloured. If undiagnosed the baby will develop liver failure and may die without a transplant. If detected within the first 6 weeks then a hepatoporto-enterostomy (Kasai procedure) can usually achieve adequate biliary drainage. Because of this it is recommended that any baby still jaundiced after 2 weeks has conjugated and unconjugated bilirubin levels checked. Those with a high conjugated fraction (>20% of total) should be referred urgently to a paediatric hepatologist for assessment.

Jaundice in older children

Jaundice is rare in older children. It is generally associated with hepatitis or with chronic liver disease. The commonest cause is hepatitis A infection. Other causes include chronic haemolysis due to hereditary spherocytosis or glucose-6-phosphate dehydrogenase (G6PD) deficiency, or liver disease such as autoimmune chronic hepatitis. Reye's syndrome, an acute encephalopathy associated with fulminant liver failure, can be induced by aspirin, and this is therefore contraindicated in young children. Deliberate paracetamol overdose is an important cause of liver failure in older children. Some inherited metabolic disorders lead to progressive jaundice. In Wilson's disease there is a defect in copper metabolism leading to neurodevelopmental delay and liver failure. Brown 'Kayser–Fleischer' rings may be visible in the cornea. Chronic hyperbilirubinaemia may be due to genetic enzyme defects such as Criggler–Najar disease (glucuronyl transferase deficiency) or abnormal hepatic uptake of bilirubin such as Gilbert's syndrome.

KEY POINTS

- Mild jaundice is extremely common in newborn infants, especially preterm babies.
- Jaundice within the first 24 hours or lasting beyond 2 weeks needs investigation.
- Phototherapy and occasionally exchange transfusion are used to treat significant jaundice.
- Biliary atresia causes an obstructive persistent jaundice with pale stools. Early treatment is essential.

Types of childhood cancer

Leukaemia
- Most common childhood malignancy (35%)
- 80% acute lymphoblastic leukaemia
- Presents with
  - malaise
  - anaemia
  - bruising
  - bone pain
  - lymphadenopathy
- Chemotherapy used to induce remission and prevent relapse
- Overall prognosis good (80% survival for acute lymphoblastic leukaemia and 70% for acute myeloid leukaemia)

Lymphoma
- Hodgkin's disease and non-Hodgkin's lymphoma (NHL)
- Usually present with lymphadenopathy
- Mediastinal lymph node involvement is common
- Diagnostic excision biopsy followed by chemotherapy

Wilms' tumour (nephroblastoma)
- Arises in mesenchymal tissue, presents as a mass
- Occasionally causes haematuria or hypertension
- Metastasize via IVC to the lungs
- 10% associated with genetic syndromes (trisomy 8, Beckwith–Wiederman syndrome or aniridia (absent iris, coded for on chromosome 11)
- 2% have abnormalities of genitourinary tract

Rhabdomyosarcoma
- Arises in mesenchymal tissue, presents as a mass
- Head and neck and genitourinary tract are the most common sites
- 15% present with metastases
- 5-year survival 70% with optimal treatment

Retinoblastoma
- Rare but important cause of blindness
- Presents within the early years
- White pupillary reflex or squint
- Most common tumour in infancy
- Cure rate 98%

Germ cell tumours
- Sacrococcygeal tumour
- Gonadal tumours
- 90% 5 year survival

Brain tumours
- Second most common presentation of childhood cancer (25%)
- Usually primary brain tumour
- Present with raised intracranial pressure or neurological signs:
  - headache
  - nausea and vomiting
  - blurred vision
  - squint (VI nerve palsy)
  - ataxia, clumsiness
  - head tilt
  - endocrine dysfunction
- Most tumours occur in the brainstem or cerebellum
- Treatment involves neurosurgical resection, chemotherapy and/or radiotherapy
- Long-term sequelae include endocrine and growth problems

Neuroblastoma
- Usually in children under 5 years
- Arises in neural crest tissue (adrenal medulla and sympathetic nervous system)
- Presents with abdominal mass, skin nodules, periorbital bruising or an unwell child depending on site of disease
- Increase in urinary catecholamine metabolites

Bone tumours
- Usually occur in older children
- Present with bone pain or mass, usually in the long bones
- Ewing's sarcoma– a primitive neuroectodermal tumour (PNET). Associated with translocations at chromosome 11 and 22; 65% 5-year survival
- Osteosarcoma— most common primary bone tumour in childhood; 65% 5 year survival,
- Treatment involves chemotherapy and surgery with bone prostheses

Management of childhood cancer

- **Diagnosis**
  The diagnosis needs to be considered in a wide range of illness presentations. Children should be referred to specialized paediatric oncology centres.
  Treatment
- The aim of treatment is eradication of the cancer, whilst minimizing damage to the normal tissues. Cancer therapy is toxic and the child requires intensive support treatment including prophylactic antibiotics and good nutritional support
  - **Surgery** is often required for diagnostic biopsy and excision of solid tumours, and for inserting indwelling central venous catheters necessary for chemotherapy and supportive care
  - **Radiotherapy** is used to treat local disease and for total body irradiation in conjunction with bone marrow transplantation. Adjacent tissues are often damaged and there may be long-term effects on growth if the spine or hypothalamo-pituitary axis is irradiated
  - **Chemotherapy** acts by killing cells during cell division. The aim is to kill the rapidly dividing malignant cells without killing normal cells. The drugs are usually given in combination at regular intervals. Side effects include hair loss, nausea, immunosuppression and bone marrow suppression. There is a particular risk of sepsis if the child becomes neutropenic, and any febrile episodes while the child is neutropenic should be treated aggressively with broad-spectrum antibiotics pending the results of blood and other cultures
  - **Bone marrow transplantation** involves either harvesting bone marrow or using compatible donated bone marrow to replace the patient's suppressed marrow; this allows more intensive chemotherapy to be used. Side effects include severe immunosuppression and graft-versus-host disease

Malignant disease affects about 1 in 600 people during childhood (1 per 10 000 children per year). The commonest malignancies are acute leukaemia and central nervous system (CNS) tumours. Overall, there has been a significant improvement in prognosis over recent years due to the use of well-researched and standardized chemotherapy regimes delivered in specialized paediatric oncology centres. The prognosis still depends largely on the particular type of malignancy and on the progression of the disease at the time of diagnosis.

Acute leukaemia

Leukaemia is the most common malignancy in childhood (30%) with an annual incidence of 3 per 100 000 children. It is due to the malignant proliferation of white cell precursors within the bone marrow. These 'blast' cells escape into the circulation and may be deposited in lymphoid or other tissue. The commonest type of leukaemia in childhood is acute lymphoblastic leukaemia (ALL), where the blast cells are precursors of lymphocytes. Chronic leukaemias are very rare in childhood.

ALL can occur at any age, but the peak is between 2 and 5 years. The prognosis is worse for those presenting under the age of 2 or over 10 years old. The onset may be insidious with malaise, anorexia and then pallor, bruising or bleeding. Lymphadenopathy and splenomegaly may be present, and bone pain may occur. Peripheral blood usually, but not always, shows anaemia, thrombocytopenia and a raised white cell count. Those with an extremely high white cell count ($>50 \times 10^9$/L) carry a worse prognosis. Blast cells may be seen on the peripheral blood film. The diagnosis is confirmed by a bone marrow aspirate, which shows the marrow infiltrated with blast cells. Cells are examined by immunophenotyping and cytogenetic analysis as these give important prognostic information. In more than 90% of cases specific genetic abnormalities can be seen in the leukaemic cell line. There may be increased numbers of chromosomes or translocations: for example, the t12:21 translocation creates a *TEL-AML1* fusion gene in 20% of children with ALL. Acute lymphoblastic leukaemia can be subdivided into common (75%), T-cell (15%), null (10%) and B-cell (1%).

Treatment of ALL involves chemotherapy to *induce* remission (i.e. remove all blast cells from the circulation and restoration of normal marrow function). Complete remission is induced in 95% of children. *Intensification* chemotherapy maintains remission, and methotrexate or cranial irradiation protects the CNS from involvement. Monthly cycles of *maintenance* chemotherapy are then required. Children who relapse are often offered high-dose chemotherapy and bone marrow transplantation. The overall prognosis for acute leukaemia is good, with up to 80% survival.

Short-term side effects of treatment

Tumour lysis syndrome

The breakdown of large numbers of malignant cells either before or during treatment can lead to very high serum urate, phosphate and potassium levels. Urate crystals can precipitate in the kidneys causing renal failure. Tumour lysis syndrome can be prevented by good hydration and the use of allopurinol (a xanthine oxidase inhibitor) or uric acid oxidase.

Bone marrow suppression and febrile neutropenia

Bone marrow suppression may be due to invasion by tumour cells or the effect of chemotherapy. Anaemia and thrombocytopenia can be treated with infusions of red cells and platelets. Neutropenia (neutrophil count $<1.0 \times 10^9$) is difficult to treat and means the patient is at risk of serious infection. Consequently any significant fever or signs and symptoms of infection while neutropenic should be investigated and treated aggressively with broad-spectrum antibiotics until culture results are known.

Immunosuppression

Severe immunosuppression may result from treatment. This leaves the child at risk from normally trivial infections. Patients should not be given live vaccines and if exposed to varicella (chickenpox) they should be given specific immunoglobulin. If the patient goes on to develop chickenpox they should be treated with aciclovir and immunoglobulin.

Nutrition

Inflammation and disruption of gut mucosa and mouth ulcers as well as anorexia can lead to poor calorie intake. Nutritional support with food supplements may be necessary.

Late sequelae of treatment

Short stature or asymmetrical growth may be caused by radiotherapy to the spine or hypothalamo-pituitary axis. The latter may also cause delayed puberty and other endocrine dysfunction including growth hormone deficiency, hypothyroidism, cortisol deficiency and gonadal failure. Cranial irradiation, especially in very young children, can lead to neurocognitive effects such as memory loss and poor attention and for this reason intensive chemotherapy and intrathecal treatment is used in some centres as an alternative. Chemotherapy can lead to subfertility, nephrotoxicity, deafness, pulmonary fibrosis and cardiomyopathy. There is a significant risk (about 12%) of second cancers due to the carcinogenic effect of chemo- and radiotherapy and an increased genetic tendency. Chronic ill health and poor school attendance may have long-term effects on educational achievement, although this may be minimized by good liaison with school and specialist staff.

KEY POINTS

- ALL is the commonest childhood malignancy, but with effective treatment the 5-year survival is in excess of 80%.
- Immunosuppression and neutropenia secondary to chemotherapy increase the risk of infection. Suspected infection must be treated aggressively.
- Survivors of childhood cancer may suffer long-term effects including poor growth and endocrine dysfunction.

Desquamation
- Loss of epidermal cells producing scaly eruption
- Examples: post scarlet fever, Kawasaki's disease

Maculopapular
- Mixture of macules and papules
- Tend to be confluent
- Examples: measles, drug rash

Vesicles
- Raised fluid-filled lesions <0.5 cm in diameter
- Bullae are large vesicles
- Example: chickenpox

Wheals
- Raised lesions with a flat top and pale centre
- Example: urticaria

Papules
- Solid palpable projections above skin surface
- Example: insect bite

Purpura and petechiae
- Purple lesions caused by small haemorrhages in the skin
- Do not fade on pressure
- Petechiae are tiny purpura
- Examples: meningococcaemia, ITP, HSP, leukaemia

Macules
- Flat pink lesions
- Examples: rubella, roseola, café-au-lait spot

What you need from your evaluation

History
- Is the child ill or febrile?
- How long has the rash or skin lesion been present?
- Could it be an insect bite or allergic reaction?
- Is it a recurrent problem?
- Is it itchy?
- Has there been contact with anyone else with a rash?

Physical examination

Describe the rash in the following terms:
- Raised or flat
- Crusty or scaly
- Colour
- Blanching on application of pressure (the glass test)
- Size of the lesions
- Distribution (discrete or generalized, or limited to certain sites on the body)

It is not uncommon for children to present with an unusual rash or for parents to be concerned about skin lesions or birthmarks on a child's skin. In some cases the rash will be acute, due to infection, allergy or skin irritation. In other children the skin changes may be part of a chronic condition or even a marker for a neurocutaneous syndrome such as neurofibromatosis or tuberous sclerosis. In babies, skin lesions may be due to congenital naevi.

While the diagnosis of skin lesions often depends on pattern recognition and having seen similar lesions before, it is important to approach this problem with a systematic, logical approach. It is also important to be able to describe the lesions appropriately, either when seeking second opinions (e.g.from a dermatologist) or consulting databases and textbooks to establish the diagnosis. Following a systematic approach is likely to reveal the diagnosis and prevent the need for requesting further investigations or causing unnecessary anxiety.

Vascular birthmarks

Capillary haemangioma
- Very common, especially in preterm infants
- Bright red lumpy lesion due to proliferation of blood vessels
- Enlarges until age 2–4 years then regresses
- Usually resolves spontaneously with no treatment
- If near important structures (airway, eyes), injection with steroid may speed regression
- Treatment – propanolol

Capillary malformation
- Sharply circumscribed, pink to purple lesion
- Present from birth (3 in 1000 births)
- Abnormal dilatation of normal dermal capillaries
- May be a sign of Sturge–Weber syndrome with an underlying meningeal haemangioma, intracranial calcification and fits
- Do not resolve but some lesions may be improved with laser therapy

Mongolian blue spot
- Blue/grey lesions in the sacral area
- More common in racial groups with pigmented skin
- Fade during the early years
- Can be confused with bruises

Pigmentation disorders

Pigmented naevus
- Can be present from birth (congenital naevus) or appear during childhood (moles)
- Contains melanocytes
- May require surgical excision if large
- If large, at risk of malignant change

Café au lait*
- May develop increasing size and number through childhood
- Seen in genetic conditions
- Neurofibromatosis
- McCune–Albright syndrome
- Links with neurological and skeletal problems

Depigmentation
- Depigmented skin patches seen in genetic disorder tuberous sclerosis
- May develop brain abnormalities, epilepsy, learning difficulties

Common transient neonatal rashes

Erythema toxicum neonatorum
- Commonest rash in newborns
- Small erythematous macules
- +/- central small pustules
- Resolves over a few days

Milia
- Very common
- Tiny epidermal cysts
- 1-2mm white/yellow popular spots
- Usually on nose, cheeks, chin, forehead
- Resolve

Miliaria*
- Occlusion of sweat ducts
- More common in hot humid environment
- Miliaria rubra usually at 10-15 days of age
- Resolves with reduced temperature

Nappy rash

Ammoniacal dermatitis
- Erythematous or papulovesicular lesions, fissures and erosions
- Skin folds spared
- Caused by irritation from excretions and chemicals
- Unusual with modern disposable nappies
- Secondary bacterial and candidal infection common, and limited use of hydrocortisone and nystatin cream. Treat by regular washing and changing, exposure to air, and use of protective creams

Candidal nappy rash
- Bright red rash with clearly demarcated edge
- Satellite lesions beyond border
- Inguinal folds usually involved
- May have oral thrush (white plaques in mouth)
- Treatment with nystatin cream, and orally if necessary

Seborrhoeic nappy rash
- Pink, greasy lesions with yellow scale
- Often in skin folds
- Cradle cap may be present
- Treat with mild topical corticosteriods

Psoriatic nappy rash
- Appearance similar to seborrhoeic dermatitis
- Family history of psoriasis

Staphylococcal scalded skin syndrome*
- Usually triggered by staphylococcal infection
- Can cause systemic illness of shock symptoms
- Swab skin to confirm infection and sensitivity
- Treat with intravenous antibiotics and systemic support measures

Scarlet fever
- Group A streptococcus tonsillitis
- Erythematous rash, sandpaper-like skin
- Pale around lips
- Inflamed tongue, strawberry appearance
- Risk of sequelae of glomerulonephritis and rheumatic fever
Treat with penicillin

► Meningococcal septicaemia
- Rapid onset septicaemia +/- meningitis
- Commonly due to meningococcus B, or C (other forms also seen)
- Vaccination for meningococcus C has reduced rate of infection
- Evolves with purple (purpuric) rash that does not blanch with pressure
- Severe septicaemic shock, coma and death within hours
- Immediate treament with antibiotic and fluid resuscitation

Chickenpox
- Very common childhood infection
- Onset 14-17 days after exposure
- Fever then rash (macule, vesicle, crusting)
- Sometimes see mucosal involvement (mouth, genitalia)
- Complications of pneumonia, secondary infection, encephalitis
- Treat symptomatically in healthy children without complications
- Immunosuppressed children at risk of severe complications
- Treat with zoster immune globulin after exposure, and aciclovir if signs of infection develop

Measles
- Rare in immunized population (MMR vaccine protects)
- Onset 10-14 days post exposure
- Morbilliform rash
- Cough, fever, conjunctivitis, irritability
- Koplick's spots (white spots in mouth)
- Rare complication of encephalitis

Rubella
- Rare in immunized population (MMR vaccine protects)
- Onset 14-21 days after exposure
- Pale morbilliform rash moves down body
- Severe fetal anomalies if mother develops rubella in first trimester

Fifth disease
- Mild illness with low-grade fever
- Slapped cheek appearance
- Lace-like rash on body
- Lasts up to 6 weeks
- Parvovirus B19 infection

Molluscum contagiosum

- Pearly dome-shaped papules with central umbilicus
- Particularly on face, axillae, neck and thighs
- Self-limited disease
- Due to molluscipox virus infection
- 'Kissing lesions' occur on opposing skin surfaces, e.g. under arms and on chest

Tinea corporis (ringworm)

- Dry, scaly papule which spreads centrifugally with central clearing
- Diagnosis confirmed microscopically by scrapings in a potassium hydroxide wet mount
- Treat with topical antifungal agents for 2–4 weeks

Impetigo

- Sticky, heaped-up, honey-coloured crusts
- Group A haemolytic streptococci or staphylococci
- Highly infectious
- Treat with antibiotics (flucloxacillin or erythromycin orally, or antibiotic cream if <5 lesions)

Cold sore

- Single or grouped vesicles or pustules sited periorally
- Recurrent herpes simplex infection
- Recur with colds and stress
- May be treated with aciclovir

Scabies

- Wheals, papules and vesicles with superimposed eczema
- Intensely itchy
- Characteristic lesion is the mite burrow between the fingers
- Head, neck, palms and soles are spared in children but not babies
- Mites can be seen on scrapings
- Treat all the household with scabicides and launder bedding

Common warts

- Roughened keratotic lesions with an irregular surface
- Occur on hands, face, knees and elbows
- Called verrucas if present on feet
- Transferred by direct contact
- Disappear spontaneously, but can be treated with salicylic acid or liquid nitrogen

Head lice (pediculosis capitis)

- Very common in schools—affects clean hair as well as dirty
- Itchy scalp
- Nits (the eggs) are visible as white specks on hair shafts
- Transmitted on clothing, combs or by direct contact
- Treated by regularly combing out the eggs using an extra fine comb or the use of anti-pediculosis shampoos. Resistance to these agents is increasing

* Courtesy of Prof John Harper. Textbook of Paediatric Dermatology, 2nd Ed, 2005. Blackwell Publishing Ltd

Atopic dermatitis (eczema)

- Erythema, wet 'weeping' areas, dry scaly, thickened skin
- Intensely itchy
- Risk of secondary bacterial (staphylococcal) and viral (herpes zoster) infection
- Often linked with other atopic problems, e.g. asthma and hay fever
- Some cases linked with food and environmental allergens
- Breast-feeding may reduce risk of eczema
- Treat with moisturizing creams to prevent skin drying
- Cream (water based) to wet areas
- Ointment (oil based) to dry areas
- Wet wraps to prevent drying and reduce scratching
- Topical steroids to persistent inflamed areas
- Topical (tacrolimus) and oral (ciclosporin) immunomodulators if severe
- Family support and follow-up important for chronic condition

Seborrhoeic dermatitis

- Dry, scaly and erythematous
- Cradle cap in infancy
- Affects face, neck, axillae and nappy area
- May look like psoriasis

Contact dermatitis

- Erythema and weeping
- Itching
- Caused by irritants such as saliva, detergents and synthetic shoes
- Looks like atopic dermatitis

Psoriasis

- Erythematous plaques
- Silver/white scales
- Extensor surfaces—scalp, knees, elbows
- Guttate psoriasis—linked to streptococcal tonsillitis (antibiotic may improve skin)
- Pitting of nail bed
- Guttate psoriasis—multiple tiny psoriatic plaques over large area of body
- Treat with topical vitamin D analogues (calcipotriol), coal tar

Henoch–Schönlein purpura

- Vasculitic illness of uncertain aetiology, often follows viral illness
- Purpuric rash to buttocks and legs
- +/- Arthritis
- +/- Abdominal pain with gastrointestinal vasculitis, risk of intussusception
- +/- Nephritis (haematuria, proteinuria, hypertension) rarely renal failure
- Some evidence steroid helpful if abdominal pain severe

Acne*

- Very common at puberty
- Linked to androgen hormones
- Pustular erythema to face, scalp and trunk
- Treat with antibiotic erythromycin or tetracyclines (over age 12)
- Hormonal treatment with antiandrogen sometimes used
- Isotretinoin for severe cases under dermatology

Kawasaki disease*

- Acute inflammatory systemic disorder
- Many features of infectious illness
- Fever > 5 days
- Macular erythematous rash
- Peeling skin typically at fingers and toes
- Lymphadenopathy
- Mucosal changes (cracked lips, strawberry tongue)
- Conjunctivitis
- Risk of coronary artery aneurysms
- Treat with immunoglobulin and aspirin

Urticaria (see Chapter 54)

* Courtesy of Prof John Harper. Textbook of Paediatric Dermatology, 2nd Ed, 2005. Blackwell Publishing Ltd.

The allergic child

Atopy
- Presents at different ages:
  Eczema—infants and preschool
  Food allergy – toddlers and preschool
  Asthma—young children
  Hay fever—teenagers
- Affects up to 1/3rd of people at some point
- Small proportion develop anaphylaxis
- Usually type I IgE mediated reaction to common allergens
- Often family history of atopy
- Breast-feeding may be protective
- Parental education and environmental adjustments may be needed

► Asthma (see Chapter 26)
- Increasing prevalence—up to 11% children
- Recurrent bronchospasm
- Cough and wheeze
- Can be life threatening—status asthmaticus
- Environmental triggers - triggers, e.g. house dust mite
- Requires bronchodilators

Food intolerance
- Non-allergic aetiology
- May be due to enzyme deficiency (e.g. lactase deficiency leading to lactose intolerance)
- Sensitivity to food additives e.g. monosodium glutamate
- Presents with colicky abdominal pain and diarrhoea
- Treat by food avoidance

Allergic conjunctivitis
- Itchy, inflamed conjunctivae with tears
- Environmental triggers similar to allergic rhinitis
- Treat with topical anti-inflammatory agents such as sodium cromoglicate drops or topical antihistamines

Hay fever (allergic rhinitis)
- 10–15% of population
- Commonly presents in adolescence
- Due to environmental triggers such as grass and tree pollens (most common in the summer months) or house dust mite (all year round)
- Sneezing, rhinitis, nasal congestion and sinusitis
- May develop nasal polyps
- Treat with antihistamines and topical corticosteroid

► Anaphylaxis
- Rapid onset of severe systemic reaction to various allergens
- Specific IgE triggers histamine release from mast cells
- Angioedema and bronchospasm can compromise breathing causing hypoxia
- Capillary leak can lead to shock
- Triggers:
  - Foods e.g. peanuts, tree nuts, fish, eggs and milk
  - Insects e.g. bees, wasps
  - Drugs e.g. antibiotics
  - Environment e.g. severe latex allergy
- Treatment with antihistamine, steroid and intramuscular adrenaline

► Eczema (see Chapter 53)
- Atopic dermatitis
- Common in infancy—extensor surfaces
- Localizes to flexoral creases in older children
- May be triggered by diet (e.g. cow's milk protein allergy) or environmental exposure (e.g. detergents)
- Treat with emollients and topical steroids

Contact dermatitis
- Type IV reaction
- Contact with nickel in cheap jewellery
- Photosensitivity rashes may be triggered by contact with certain plants
- Skin patch testing may be helpful in identifying cause

What you need from your evaluation

History
- Is there a family history of atopy (hay fever, eczema or asthma)?
- Did the child have eczema during infancy?
- Is there an obvious environmental trigger?
- Take a full dietary history—keeping an allergy diary may help identify the cause
- What allergen avoidance has been tried so far?
- Ask about drugs—is there a history of drug allergy?
- What treatments have been needed in the past?—previous need for adrenaline shows the allergy may be life threatening
- How much is the child's daily life affected by their allergies?

Examination
- **Airway:** is there any evidence of stridor or significant angioedema of the lips or tongue? Is there nasal congestion or polyps?
- **Breathing:** observe for signs of respiratory distress and check for wheeze. Beware the 'silent chest' of severe status asthmaticus
- **Circulation:** check capillary refill for evidence of shock. Blood pressure should be measured, but hypotension is a very late sign
- **Skin:** check for urticaria (wheals), excoriation and vesicles of eczema. Lichenification suggests chronic severe eczema

Investigations
- Check for specific IgE antibodies to suspected allergens, e.g. tree pollen, peanut, milk, egg, house dust mite
- Skin prick testing may be helpful in contact dermatitis but has poor specificity—a positive test may indicate sensitization but does not necessarily correlate with symptoms
- PEFR and lung function tests in asthma, including reversibility test after bronchodilator treatment
- Controlled allergen challenge—a carefully controlled exposure to increasing quantities of allergen to test whether allergy has persisted after a period of exclusion. Must be undertaken with care, and with facilities for emergency treatment of anaphylaxis

Atopic disease

Allergy is one of the most common childhood diseases, affecting more than 1 in 4 children at some point. The incidence seems to be increasing in many countries worldwide, and the reason is not clear. Exposure to pollutants may be one factor; over-cleanliness and lack of exposure to infections and allergens in early life may be another.

Allergy is caused when an individual develops IgE antibody against specific environmental allergens. Once sensitized, an atopic individual will trigger a type I (immediate) hypersensitivity response on exposure to the same allergen, leading to local or systemic inflammation. This inflammation is mediated by release of histamine and other cytokines from mast cells, and leads to:
- Acute inflammation (urticaria)
- Bronchospasm (asthma)
- Chronic inflammation (e.g. eczema).

Life-threatening airway obstruction (angioedema) or shock may occur if there is a massive systemic response to allergen exposure (anaphylaxis).

The age of onset is variable, but most atopic children develop symptoms by 5 or 6 years of age. Infants are likely to show eczema and milk or egg allergy. Preschool children tend to get asthma, initially triggered by viral infection and later by environmental allergens such as house dust mite. Allergic rhinitis and conjunctivitis are commoner in older children and young adults. A family history of atopy is often present. There is good evidence that prolonged exclusive breastfeeding reduces later allergy.

Eczema

Eczema is discussed in detail in Chapter.

Asthma

Acute asthma is discussed in Chapter. Chronic asthma management is discussed in Chapter 26.

Allergic rhinitis

Allergic rhinitis (hay fever) reaches a peak in adolescence. Sneezing, rhinorrhoea, nasal congestion and itching are triggered by an IgE response to airborne allergens. Tree and grass pollens, mould spores and pet dander are common triggers. Pollens are particularly prevalent in early summer on dry, hot days. The child may exhibit the 'allergic salute' of rubbing their nose constantly with their hand. Nasal polyps can develop with chronic inflammation. Treatment involves antihistamines and nasal topical steroid.

Allergic conjunctivitis

Many children with allergic rhinitis will also have recurrent non-infective conjunctivitis; the eyes are red, feel gritty and itchy and tearful. Treatment involves topical antihistamines or topical mast cell stabilizers such as sodium cromoglicate.

Food allergy

Food allergy is IgE mediated and appears to be increasing, affecting 3–6% of preschoolers and 2–3% of school-age children. In young infants the symptoms are often cutaneous, with eczema, urticaria, and angioedema. Wheeze, diarrhoea or vomiting may be present. Colic occurs in babies. In infants and toddlers the commonest food allergens are cow's milk protein, egg and peanuts. There is cross-reactivity (30%) between cow's milk protein allergy and soya milk allergy. In older children reactions to citrus fruits, tree nuts or peanuts, fish or shellfish are more common.

The diagnosis is made on the basis of a clear history of exposure, the presence of significant specific IgE antibody or a positive skin prick test, and preferably confirmed by a standardized controlled food challenge. Treatment involves excluding the allergen from the diet, usually for a period of 2 years, and then a controlled food challenge. A dietician should advise on maintaining a balanced diet (e.g. calcium supplements if milk is excluded). Severe anaphylaxis is relatively rare and there is a danger of over-diagnosis leading to a very restricted diet and lifestyle. Children with concurrent asthma are at most risk and may need to carry adrenaline and wear a Medic-Alert bracelet. Very rarely there may be cross-reactivity between airborne allergens and food allergens (e.g. birch pollen and apples) leading to seasonal mucosal inflammation in response to certain foods (oral allergy syndrome).

Food *sensitivity* is not IgE mediated and causes predominantly gastrointestinal symptoms, such as abdominal pain, vomiting, diarrhoea and colitis.

Urticaria, angioedema and anaphylaxis

A variety of allergens including foods, insect stings and drugs may cause a severe acute allergic reaction. At its most extreme and life-threatening this is known as anaphylaxis. Many allergic reactions will start with an urticarial rash—raised, well demarcated itchy wheals with an erythematous border and a pale centre (see Chapter). In a few cases urticaria may non-allergic, triggered by mast cells releasing histamine in response to cold, pressure (the Koebner phenomenon), or other physical causes. Contact dermatitis (a delayed or type IV IgE-mediated reaction) also causes urticaria. Angioedema is acute tissue swelling around the eyes, lips or airway in response to an immediate type I IgE reaction. This may cause stridor and airway obstruction.

Anaphylaxis involves massive release of inflammatory mediators causing systemic inflammation and shock due to vasodilatation and capillary leak. Airway obstruction due to oedema and bronchospasm may occur. There is a very rapid onset of symptoms, often associated with flushing, tachycardia and a feeling of 'impending doom'. Common triggers include drugs (e.g. penicillins, anaesthetic agents), foods (peanuts, shellfish), latex (in rubber gloves) and insect stings (wasps, bees). Treatment includes removal of the allergen, intramuscular adrenaline, oral antihistamines and intravenous hydrocortisone.

Patients with a history of anaphylaxis should be referred to an allergy clinic for specialist management. It may be appropriate to provide the child with an adrenaline auto-injector (e.g. Epipen) which can be used to administer a fixed dose of adrenaline intramuscularly at the onset of symptoms. Preventative advice to the child, their parents and school or nursery is critical, though should not over-restrict lifestyle.

KEY POINTS

- The incidence of atopy is increasing in industrialized countries.
- Eczema and milk allergy are common in infancy but normally resolve.
- Seasonal allergic rhinitis and conjunctivitis are common (up to 40% of teenagers)
- Testing for allergy is controversial as skin prick tests and IgE assays may be equivocal.
- Prevention by education and allergen avoidance is crucial for all atopic conditions.
- Severe anaphylaxis to foods is rare, but does cause a few preventable deaths each year.

Presentation of the acutely ill child

Children may become critically ill very rapidly and their survival depends on prompt recognition of the severity of their illness, appropriate life support and rapid treatment. Parents are usually able to recognize that their child is acutely unwell, even if they are not able to pinpoint the exact cause. Worried parents will often take their children to a primary care centre or present to an emergency department for an urgent medical opinion

Recognition of acute illness

It is very important that health professionals are able to rapidly identify signs of serious illness and triage children appropriately for further investigation and treatment. Fever is a very common presentation of infectious diseases and identifying warning signs or 'red flags' is important. The table below lists some features that should alert you to the severity of an acute illness:

Common presentations of an acutely unwell child

- High fever, often of sudden onset (Chapter 21)
- A non-blanching rash (septicaemia)
- Altered level of consciousness (Chapter 40)
- Severe dehydration
- Convulsions
- Anaphylaxis
- Inhaled foreign body or choking
- Acute asthma attack
- Drug ingestion (accidental or deliberate)
- Burns and scalds

If early signs of acute illness are missed the child may eventually progress to a cardio-respiratory arrest (see Chapter 56). In children cardiac arrest usually follows respiratory or circulatory failure rather than being due to a primary cardiac problem. By recognizing these signs and treating them urgently cardiac arrest is often preventable

	Green—low risk	Amber—intermediate risk	Red—high risk
Colour	• Normal colour of skin, lips and tongue	• Pallor reported by parent/carer	• Pale/mottled/ashen/blue
Activity	• Responds normally to social cues • Content/smiles • Stays awake or awakens quickly • Strong normal cry/not crying	• Not responding normally to social cues • Wakes only with prolonged stimulation • Decreased activity • No smile	• No response to social cues • Appears ill to a healthcare professional • Does not wake or if roused does not stay awake • Weak, high-pitched or continuous
Respiratory		• Nasal flaring • Tachyponea: – RR>50 breaths/min, age 6–12 months – RR>40 breaths/min, age >12 months • Oxygen saturation <95% in air • Crackles	• Grunting • Tachypnoea: – RR>60 breaths/min • Moderate or severe chest chest indrawing
Hydration	• Normal skin and eyes • Moist mucous membranes	• Dry mucous membranes • Poor feeding in infants • CRT ≥3 seconds • Reduced urine output	• Reduced skin turgor
Other	• None of the amber or red symptoms or signs	• Fever for ≥5 days	• Age 0–3 months, temp. ≥ 38°C • Age 3–6 months, temp. ≥ 39°C
		• Swelling of a limb or joint • Non-weight bearing/ not using an extremity	• Non-blanching rash • Bulging fontanelle • Neck stiffness • Status epilepticus • Focal neurological signs • Focal seizures
		• A new lump >2 cm	• Bile-stained vomiting

(Table from NICE guideline on feverish illness in children)

Fluid loss
- Blood loss
- ►Vomiting
- Diarrhoea
- Burns

Fluid maldistribution
- ►Septic shock
- Cardiac disease
- ►Anaphylaxis
- Nephrotic syndrome (capillary leak)

Respiratory distress
- Foreign body
- Croup
- ►Asthma
- ►Bronchiolitis
- Pneumonia

Respiratory depression
- Convulsions
- Raised ICP
- ►Poisoning
- Opiates

CIRCULATORY FAILURE (SHOCK)

RESPIRATORY FAILURE

CARDIAC ARREST

Circulatory failure (shock)

Shock is used to describe a state of inadequate tissue perfusion due to an acute failure of circulation. The body responds by redistributing blood to vital organs such as the brain and the heart, at the expense of the skin, muscles and bowel. Children in shock look pale and have poor skin perfusion. Blood pressure is maintained in children by peripheral vasoconstriction, so that hypotension is a very late sign of shock. Capillary refill time, checked centrally, is a more reliable sign of circulatory failure. Normal is a capillary refill within 2 seconds

Fluid loss: dehydration

Anaphylaxis

Heart failure

Blood loss

Fluid loss:
• Diabetic ketoacidosis

Septic shock:
• Meningococcal septicaemia
• Toxic shock syndrome

Fluid loss: burns

Clinical features of shock
• Tachycardia
• Thready pulse
• Delayed capillary refill
• Mottled, pale skin
• Cool extremities
• Hypotension (late sign)
• Tachypnoea
• Restlessness
• Reduced urine output
• Metabolic acidosis

Signs that suggest cause
• Fever in sepsis
• Purpuric rash (meningococcus)
• Hepatomegaly (heart failure)
• Focus of infection

Management
• High flow oxygen, respiratory support
• Intravenous fluid bolus
• Consider inotropic support
• Antibiotics for septic shock
• Adrenaline (epinephrine) and hydrocortisone for anaphylaxis

Causes of respiratory failure

Upper airway obstruction
• Foreign body
• Epiglottitis
• Croup
• Loss of pharyngeal tone
• Flexion or hyperextension of neck

Neurological
• Head injury
• Meningitis
• Raised ICP
• Muscle weakness

Lower airway
• Asthma
• Bronchiolitis
• Pneumonia
• Cystic fibrosis
• Neonatal lung disease

Severe cardiac failure

Drug ingestion

Clinical features
• Shortness of breath
• Tachypnoea
• Cyanosis
• Nasal flaring
• Grunting
• Intercostal recession
• Restlessness or confusion

Symptoms and signs of the underlying disease
• Expiratory wheeze
• Inspiratory stridor
• Crackles
• Neurological weakness

Management
• Assess severity by examination, blood gases and oxygen saturation monitor
• Give high flow oxygen
• Intubate and ventilate if rising P_{CO_2}. (The decision to ventilate is based on clinical criteria, not just blood gases)
• Treat the underlying cause: antibiotics (infection), bronchodilators and steroids (asthma), remove foreign body

Investigations
• Oxygen saturation
• Arterial blood gases
• Chest radiograph

Respiratory failure

Respiratory failure is defined as inadequate respiration to maintain normal arterial oxygen and carbon dioxide concentrations. Respiratory failure is obvious if the child is apnoeic or deeply cyanosed, but it is important to be able to detect impending respiratory failure and to intervene quickly. Tachypnoea >50/min, grunting and oxygen saturation <95% are signs of serious respiratory distress.

Acute upper airway obstruction

Acute upper airway obstruction is a medical emergency. It can be due to infection (epiglottitis, croup) or inhalation of a foreign body (especially common in toddlers who put small objects in their mouths). Presentation is with acute sudden onset of choking, coughing and cyanosis, followed by collapse. There may be an inspiratory stridor (see Chapter 24) and marked intercostal recession. If epiglottitis is suspected do not examine the child's throat. The management of choking is described in Chapter 56.

Septic shock

Meningococcal septicaemia is one of the most life-threatening causes of septic shock and is due to Gram-negative diplocccus *Neisseria meningitides* infection. 40–50% will present with meningitis (see Chapter 57), 40% with meningitis and septicaemia and 10% with septicaemia alone. Within hours of the onset of non-specific flu-like symptoms, a rash develops. This may initially be erythematous or petechial but rapidly becomes purpuric. Parents are advised to perform the 'glass test' (pressing on the skin with a glass beaker—see Chapter 52) to check whether any rash is non-blanching and seek urgent medical advice if positive.

Meningococcal disease should be suspected if there is:
- Fever and a non-blanching rash, especially if also
- The child looks ill
- The non-blanching lesions are >2 mm (purpura)
- There is neck stiffness
- The capillary refill time is ≥3 seconds.

Fulminant septicaemia can develop within hours, leading to endotoxin-mediated severe septic shock and coma. The case fatality rate is around 10%. Any child with purpura and a fever should be given intramusular ceftriaxone and transferred to hospital immediately. The meningococcus C vaccine does not protect against the more common B strain. As 20–30% of the population may be nasopharyngeal carriers of *Neisseria meningitides*, close contacts should be given rifampicin prophylaxis.

Staphylococcal toxic shock syndrome presents very acutely with high fever, muscle pain, a desquamating rash and severe circulatory failure. It is mediated by *Staphyloccocus aureus* exotoxins. The original site of infection may be trivial, such as a graze, or in girls may be associated with menstruation. Circulatory support and high-dose antibiotic treatment with flucloxacillin or clindamycin is required.

Neurological warning signs

Signs of an actual or impending serious neurological disorder include
- Drowsiness, lethargy or other altered level of consciousness
- Severe headache, especially if associated with vomiting
- Irritability or a high-pitched cry
- Bulging fontanelle (infants)
- Neck stiffness
- Sudden onset of muscle weakness
- Any new cranial nerve lesion
- Abnormal movements
- Convulsions

These signs should prompt a thorough search for the cause. Consider raised intracranial pressure, central nervous system (CNS) infection and whether neuroimaging with CT or MRI scan is required.

KEY POINTS

- Early recognition of impending cardiorespiratory failure is vital.
- Irritability may be an early sign of hypoxia or CNS infection.
- A non-blanching rash in an ill child should be assumed to be meningococcal septicaemia and is a medical emergency.

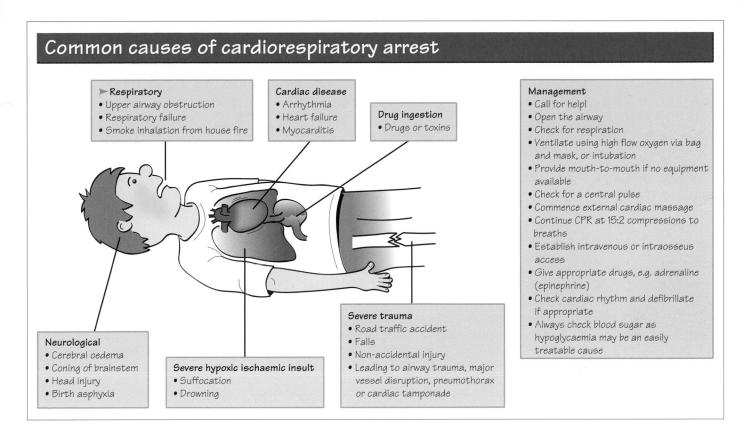

Common causes of cardiorespiratory arrest

▶Respiratory
- Upper airway obstruction
- Respiratory failure
- Smoke inhalation from house fire

Cardiac disease
- Arrhythmia
- Heart failure
- Myocarditis

Drug ingestion
- Drugs or toxins

Management
- Call for help!
- Open the airway
- Check for respiration
- Ventilate using high flow oxygen via bag and mask, or intubation
- Provide mouth-to-mouth if no equipment available
- Check for a central pulse
- Commence external cardiac massage
- Continue CPR at 15:2 compressions to breaths
- Establish intravenous or intraosseus access
- Give appropriate drugs, e.g. adrenaline (epinephrine)
- Check cardiac rhythm and defibrillate if appropriate
- Always check blood sugar as hypoglycaemia may be an easily treatable cause

Neurological
- Cerebral oedema
- Coning of brainstem
- Head injury
- Birth asphyxia

Severe hypoxic ischaemic insult
- Suffocation
- Drowning

Severe trauma
- Road traffic accident
- Falls
- Non-accidental injury
- Leading to airway trauma, major vessel disruption, pneumothorax or cardiac tamponade

Collapse and cardiorespiratory arrest

Not all children who collapse will proceed to a full respiratory or cardiac arrest. Causes of sudden collapse in children are listed in the box and many of these are discussed in detail in Chapters 40 and 57. However, if basic life support is not provided urgently, a collapsed child may progress to cardiorespiratory arrest, often due to failure to maintain an open airway.

Sudden collapse in children

- Syncope (vaso-vagal)
- Epilepsy
- Choking
- Cardiac arrhythmia (rare)
- Factitious illness (rare)
- Hypoglycaemia
- Drug ingestion
- Anaphylaxis

Cardiac arrest is the end-point of severe respiratory or cardiac failure that has either been overwhelming or has not been ade-quately treated. Cardiorespiratory arrest outside hospital requires rapid basic life support until skilled help arrives. In hospital, arrest should be managed by a skilled resuscitation team. As most cardiorespiratory arrests in children are secondary to hypoxia rather than due to cardiac disease it is crucial to achieve a patent airway and adequate oxygenation using high-flow oxygen and artificial respiration and where necessary (e.g. asystole or severe bradycardia) to circulate this oxygen by use of cardiac massage.

Establishing an airway and artificial ventilation

The airway should be opened by lifting the chin and tilting the head back to a 'sniffing the air' position. In infants the head should be in the neutral position. If there is a possibility of cervical spine injury then the airway should be opened by the 'jaw-thrust' method, while a helper supports the cervical spine. The airway should then be cleared by removing any vomit or secretions with suction. Artificial ventilation can be given by mouth to mouth or in infants by mouth to mouth and nose. After five rescue breaths check for signs of circulation (i.e. moving, normal breathing, coughing or presence of a central pulse). If there are no signs of life then commence cardiac massage.

Paediatrics at a Glance, Third Edition. Lawrence Miall, Mary Rudolf, Dominic Smith. © 2012 John Wiley & Sons, Ltd. Published 2012 by John Wiley & Sons, Ltd.

The correct airway position for children of different ages

Neutral position in an infant

'Sniffing the air' position in a small child (pre-puberty)

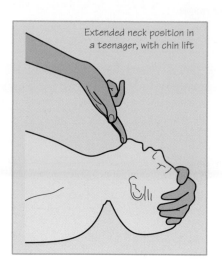

Extended neck position in a teenager, with chin lift

Choking

Children are at high risk of obstructing their airway with a foreign body. This is partly due to their nature (toddlers putting small objects in their mouths, older children throwing food in the air or sucking on pen-tops) and partly due to the small size of the airway and the anatomy. A child's airway is conical, with the narrowest part at the cricoid ring, so objects tend to lodge in a position where they can cause complete airway obstruction. This leads to sudden onset of choking, cyanosis and collapse. Choking should be managed by encouraging coughing or in the unconscious child by opening the airway, removing any visible obstruction and performing alternating back blows and chest/abdominal thrusts to expel the obstruction. Abdominal thrusts (the Heimlich manoeuvre) should not be attempted in infants because of the risk of trauma to the liver and spleen; instead, perform five alternate back blows and chest thrusts with the child held in a head-down position. If these measures are unsuccessful ventilation will be required via an emergency tracheostomy or crico-thyroidotomy.

External cardiac massage

In infants cardiac massage can be achieved by encircling the chest with both hands and compressing the lower third of the sternum with the thumbs. In young children the heel of one hand is used and in older children two hands are used. A ratio of 15 compres-

Cardiac massage in (a) an infant, and (b) an older child

(a)

(b)

(a) The Heimlich manoeuvre

(b) Back blows to an infant

sions to 2 breaths is used for all ages except *newborn* infants, where the ratio is 3:1.

If these measures are not effective then drugs such as adrenaline (epinephrine), sodium bicarbonate and a fluid bolus may be necessary, depending on the cause of the cardiac arrest. Adrenaline can be given via the intravenous or intraosseous routes. Endotracheal adrenaline should only be used if intravenous or intraosseous access is impossible, as the evidence for efficacy is not good. Defibrillation is very rarely required in paediatric cardiac arrests, but is indicated for certain cardiac arrhythmias such as ventricular fibrillation, ventricular tachycardia and supraventricular tachycardia unresponsive to drug therapy. Life-threatening cardiac arrhythmias are more common in children with congenital heart disease (postoperatively), drug ingestion (e.g. overdose of a tricyclic antidepressant) and in those with a long QT interval on the ECG.

Focal points for the assessment of the collapsed child

• Call for help immediately.
• Make a rapid assessment of the child's responsiveness—stimulate and say 'are you all right?'. Do not shake the child.
• If the child responds and is breathing with an open airway, leave them in this position and await help.
• If the child does not respond and is not breathing, proceed with basic life support.
• If the child is breathing normally but not responding to you, turn them onto their side in the recovery position.

• Continue basic life support uninterrupted until help arrives. If help has not arrived after 1 minute of CPR then go and get help.
• Apply pressure to any active bleeding points.
• Rapidly assess the neurological state by looking at pupils, posture and the level of consciousness.
• Once help arrives, or if in a hospital setting:
  ○ Continue basic life support uninterrupted.
  ○ Commence advanced life support (e.g. tracheal intubation, vascular access, administration of drugs) as indicated.
  ○ Commence monitoring (ECG, oxygen saturation).
  ○ Always check blood sugar level.
• Perform appropriate investigations and commence definitive treatment (e.g. infection screen and broad spectrum antibiotics if sepsis is suspected).
• Once the child has been stabilized, transfer to an intensive care unit for definitive care.

KEY POINTS

• Cardiac arrest is usually secondary to respiratory failure or shock.
• Upper airway obstruction is a common cause of acute respiratory failure in young children.
• Opening the airway and providing adequate oxygenation is critical.
• The technique of basic life support is a practical skill which you should acquire.

Causes of coma

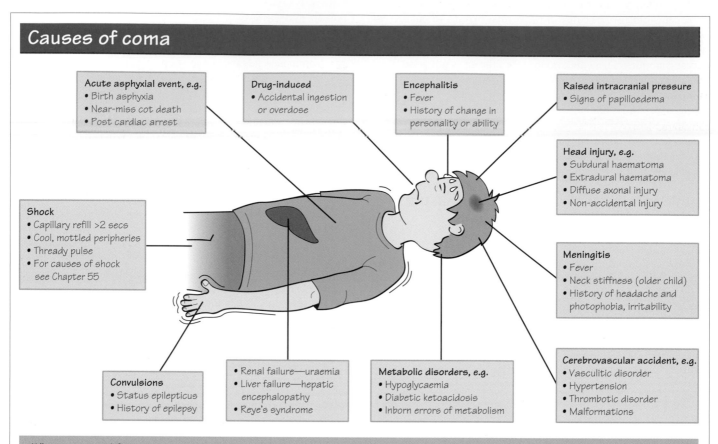

Acute asphyxial event, e.g.
- Birth asphyxia
- Near-miss cot death
- Post cardiac arrest

Drug-induced
- Accidental ingestion or overdose

Encephalitis
- Fever
- History of change in personality or ability

Raised intracranial pressure
- Signs of papilloedema

Head injury, e.g.
- Subdural haematoma
- Extradural haematoma
- Diffuse axonal injury
- Non-accidental injury

Shock
- Capillary refill >2 secs
- Cool, mottled peripheries
- Thready pulse
- For causes of shock see Chapter 55

Meningitis
- Fever
- Neck stiffness (older child)
- History of headache and photophobia, irritability

Convulsions
- Status epilepticus
- History of epilepsy

- Renal failure—uraemia
- Liver failure—hepatic encephalopathy
- Reye's syndrome

Metabolic disorders, e.g.
- Hypoglycaemia
- Diabetic ketoacidosis
- Inborn errors of metabolism

Cerebrovascular accident, e.g.
- Vasculitic disorder
- Hypertension
- Thrombotic disorder
- Malformations

What you need from your evaluation

History

- Ask about the possibility of drug ingestion (either deliberate or accidental in young children)
- Was there a prodromal illness or contact with serious infection (e.g. meningitis)
- Assess the possibility of non-accidental injury (Chapter 65 neglect and abuse)
- Is there a history of convulsions and for how long did they last?
- Was the child neuro-developmentally normal prior to the onset of coma?

Examination

- **Vital signs:** is there a bradycardia (suggests raised ICP) or tachyarrhythmia (drug ingestion). Deep, sighing (Kussmaul) respiration suggests diabetic ketoacidosis. Ketones may be smelt on the breath
- Look for a focus of infection. Check for rashes and neck stiffness, pneumonia and UTI
- Check pupils: are they symmetrical and do they constrict appropriately to light?
- Check for abnormal posture (decorticate or decerebrate posture)
- Assess the level of consciousness using either the modified Glasgow Coma Score (GCS) or the more rapid AVPU (see opposite)
- Always check the blood glucose. Hypoglycaemia is the most common metabolic cause of coma

Investigations and their significance

- Blood glucose — Hypo- or hyperglycaemia
- Full blood count — May indicate infection or acute blood loss (Hb and PCV low)
- Blood culture — May identify infective cause
- U&E — High urea in dehydration. Sodium may be high or low
- Blood gases — Metabolic or respiratory acidosis (see Chapter 5 for interpretation)
- Chest radiograph — Infection or cardiac failure, trauma (e.g. rib fracture)
- CT or MRI scan — Focal pathology (tumour, haemorrhage, abscess)
- Lumbar puncture — May show evidence of infection (meningitis, encephalitis) or bleeding (e.g. subarachnoid haemorrhage)
- Metabolic screen — Ammonia may be raised in urea cycle defects and Reye's syndrome
- LFTs — May be elevated in hepatic encephalopathy
- Urine — Toxicology screen for poisoning or overdose Ketones (DKA) and culture (sepsis)

LP should not be attempted in the unconscious child until raised ICP has been excluded, due to the risk of brain herniation (coning)

AVPU coma scale

Alert
Voice (responds to)
Pain (responds to)
Unresponsive

A score of 'P' corresponds to a GCS of 8, and suggests the airway should be protected by intubation to prevent aspiration

Coma

A child who is deeply unconscious is said to be in coma. *Encephalopathy* refers to the precomatose state with an altered conscious level. An unconscious child requires urgent and careful evaluation to establish the cause of the coma and to commence appropriate therapy. Whatever the cause the airway must be protected and adequate ventilation maintained.

Meningitis

Meningitis is caused by either bacterial or viral infection invading the membranes overlying the brain and spinal cord and should be considered in any irritable child with unexplained fever. It is commonest in the neonatal period but can occur at any age. The causes are listed in the box.

Causes of meningitis

Viral
- Mumps virus
- Coxsackie virus
- Echovirus
- Herpes simplex virus
- Poliomyelitis (if unvaccinated)

Bacterial
- *Neisseria meningitidis*
- *Streptococcus pneumoniae*
- *Haemophilus influenzae* type B (now rare if immunized)
- Group B streptococcus (in newborn)
- *Escherichia coli* and listeria (in newborn)

Viral meningitis is preceded by pharyngitis or gastrointestinal (GI) upset. The child then develops fever, headache and neck stiffness. In **bacterial meningitis** the child is drowsy and may be vacant. Irritability is a common feature, often with a high-pitched cry, and convulsions may occur. Examination shows an ill child, with a stiff neck and positive Kernig's sign (pain on extending the legs). These signs are not reliable in young infants. Tonsillitis and otitis media can also mimic neck stiffness. In infants the fontanelle may be bulging. A petechial or purpuric rash suggests meningococcal meningitis.

Meningitis is confirmed by a lumbar puncture (see Chapter 5), which shows a leucocytosis, high protein count, low glucose and may show organisms present. The fluid will look cloudy to the naked eye. Culture or PCR analysis will confirm the organism, but treatment should be commenced empirically as soon as the cultures have been taken.

Intravenous ceftriaxone is usually given, depending on the age of the child and the likely organism. Steroids reduce meningeal inflammation in haemophilus meningitis. Meninigococcal meningitis is associated with pharyngeal carriage and household contacts should receive prophylaxis with rifampicin. Meningococcal septicaemia is discussed in Chapter 52.

Encephalitis

Viral infection sometimes spreads beyond the meninges to infect the brain tissue itself. This is known as meningo-encephalitis. The onset is often more insidious and the child's personality may change or they may become confused or clumsy before the onset of coma. Meningism is less of a feature. The lumbar puncture shows a lymphocytosis and specimens should be sent for viral culture and PCR analysis. Herpes simplex virus or *Mycoplasma pneumoniae* may be responsible, so always ask about contact with herpetic lesions (cold sores). Treatment with aciclovir, erythromycin and cefotaxime is given until the organism is known.

In herpes encephalitis the EEG and an MRI brain scan may characteristically show temporal lobe involvement.

Metabolic causes of coma

In the absence of trauma or infection, a metabolic cause for coma must be considered. By far the commonest metabolic cause is hypoglycaemia, and blood glucose must be measured immediately at the bedside in every unconscious child. Hypoglycaemia may be due to inadequate carbohydrate intake or excess insulin in children with diabetes mellitus, but it can also be the presenting feature in infants with inborn errors of metabolism or adrenal insufficiency. Hyperglycaemia in uncontrolled diabetes can lead to ketoacidosis with coma, though the onset is often more gradual. Diabetes is discussed in detail in Chapter 18.

Any severe metabolic derangement can cause coma, including severe uraemia (in renal failure) or high ammonia (inborn errors of metabolism such as urea cycle disorders), severe hypernatraemia or hyponatraemia. Coma can also be caused by cerebral oedema from over-rapid correction of electrolyte imbalance in severe dehydration.

Reye's syndrome

Reye's syndrome may be preceded by a viral illness such as influenza or chickenpox, and is commoner in winter. Although it is rare and not in itself infectious it can be triggered by the use of aspirin (salicylic acid) during a viral illness and hence aspirin is not recommended in childhood. The exact aetiology is unknown, but there is an initial phase of vomiting and lethargy followed by a non-inflammatory encephalopathic illness with personality change, irritability and then coma with raised intracranial pressure. Fatty change (steatosis) in the liver may lead to acute hepatic failure. Treatment is mainly supportive with aggressive intensive care treatment to treat raised intracranial pressure.

Unexplained coma

In unexplained coma the possibility of non-accidental injury such as shaking injury must be considered. A CT brain scan and skeletal survey may show evidence of trauma and retinal haemorrhages may be present. Accidental drug ingestion or overdose, or deliberate poisoning may cause coma, and a urine toxicology screen can sometimes identify the drug. Drugs affecting the central nervous system such as opiate analgaesics, alcohol and antidepressants are often implicated.

KEY POINTS

- Evaluate coma using the AVPU (alert, voice, pain, unresponsive) score.
- Always check the blood glucose in coma.
- Consider poisoning, drug overdose or non-accidental injury.
- Altered consciousness, fever and irritability suggest meningitis, even in the absence of neck stiffness.
- Never perform a lumbar puncture in an unconscious child until raised intracranial pressure has been excluded.
- Consider Reye's syndrome if there has been ingestion of aspirin or recent viral infection.

---

58 The fitting child

Causes of convulsions

Head injury
• History of trauma
• Intracranial bleeding on CT scan

Hypoglycaemia
• Diabetes or inborn errors of metabolism
• Responds to glucose

Meningitis
• Fever and meningism
• Diagnose by lumbar puncture

Febrile convulsions
• Generalized convulsion
• Presence of high fever
• Age: 5 months to 5 years

Asphyxial injury
• Hypoxic episode (e.g. near-drowning or cardiac arrest)

Electrolyte imbalance
• Hyponatraemia
• Hypocalcaemia

Drug ingestion
• Poisoning

Epilepsy
• Check anticonvulsant compliance

What you need from your evaluation

History

● Is there a history of previous convulsions? The child may have established epilepsy
● How long has the convulsion lasted? Seizures lasting less than 20 min are unlikely to cause brain damage
● Obtain an accurate description of the convulsion—how did it begin, was it focal or generalized? Speak to witnesses. Some parents may have video footage
● Was the child unwell or pyrexial beforehand? Could it be a febrile convulsion or part of a CNS infection?
● Is the child developmentally normal? Non-febrile convulsions are much more common in children with learning disability or cerebral palsy
● Is drug ingestion or poisoning possible? There may be an organic treatable cause for the fits

Examination

● Make sure the airway is open
● Is the convulsion generalized, affecting all limbs?
● Check the temperature
● Is there an obvious focus of infection?
● Are there signs of trauma or head injury?
● Examine the eyes—are they flickering or rolling?
● Look for signs of meningitis and check the pupils

Treatment

● Give oxygen and maintain a patent airway
● Place the child in the recovery position
● Give buccal midazolam or rectal diazepam
● Correct any metabolic disturbance
● Give dextrose if hypoglycaemia likely
● Consider IV anticonvulsants—lorazepam, phenytoin, or phenobarbital
● If in prolonged status epilepticus, thiopental infusion and ventilation may be needed

Investigations and their significance

● Blood glucose — Must always be checked in any fitting child. Can be done at the bedside
● U&E, calcium, magnesium — Hyponatraemia, hypocalcaemia and hypomagnesaemia can cause fits
● Lumbar puncture — If meningitis suspected, but beware raised ICP in prolonged fit
● CT/MRI scan — If any history of trauma or focal neurological signs suggesting intracranial lesion
● Blood and urine cultures, throat swab, CXR — To look for focus of infection in febrile convulsions
● Urine toxicology — If drug ingestion or overdose suspected

Generalized convulsions

The term *convulsion* is synonymous with *fit* or *seizure*. Convulsions are due to synchronous discharge of electrical activity from a number of neurons, usually with loss of consciousness and abnormal movements. In a generalized convulsion all four limbs and the face are affected. Convulsions are common, occurring in 3–5% of children. They do not necessarily mean the child will go on to develop epilepsy, and many children only ever have one convulsion. However, 60% of epilepsy develops in childhood (Chapter 41). Children's brains are particularly susceptible to convulsions and the commonest trigger is the rise in temperature during a febrile illness.

Febrile convulsions

These occur between the ages of 6 months and 5 years in normal children and are triggered by fever, usually as part of an URTI, although they may also be triggered by any febrile illness. They can be simple or complex (see table).

Simple febrile convulsion (75%)	Complex febrile convulsion (25%)
Child age 6 months–6 years Single seizure lasting <15 min Neurologically normal before and after Normal neurodevelopment Fever not due to CNS infection	As for simple febrile convulsion but: Seizure focal or prolonged >15 min, or Many seizures occurring in close succession, or Status epilepticus

Febrile convulsions should be managed by identifying and treating the source of the fever, and cooling the child by undressing them and sponging with tepid water. Antipyretics such as paracetamol or ibuprofen should be given. If the convulsion persists for more than 10 minutes give anticonvulsants. Status epilepticus (see below) occurs in less than 1% of febrile convulsions. Investigations should be performed to exclude serious infection, and if no obvious focus of infection is found a lumbar puncture is indicated to exclude meningitis.

Advice to parents is very important. About one third of children will have further febrile convulsions in the future. Parents must be taught how to manage fever and basic first aid management of convulsions. The good prognosis should be explained. Children with uncomplicated febrile convulsions are at very little risk of. Overall the risk of epilepsy is 2–3% (about twice the normal incidence). Prophylactic anticonvulsants don't seem to reduce the risk of future convulsions. If seizures are very frequent a benzodiazepine can be given at the onset of seizure prior to transfer to hospital.

Management of the fitting child

Most parents who witness their child having a seizure imagine that the child is going to die and seek medical attention urgently. Children may still be fitting when they present. The most important thing is to support the airway and turn the child into the recovery position, semi-prone with the knee flexed under the chest and the hand under the head. Objects (other than an oropharyngeal airway) should not be put into the mouth. If oxygen is available this should be given by facemask. If the convulsion is ongoing, lorazepam should be given intravenously to terminate the seizure. If intravenous access is not possible, buccal midazolam or rectal diazepam may be used. Occasionally some convulsions persist; this is known as status epilepticus (see below).

It is vital to check blood glucose immediately in any fitting child, as hypoglycaemia is a common and rapidly treatable cause. Not all children with hypoglycaemic convulsions are diabetic; some may have inborn errors of metabolism. Once the convulsion has terminated the child may remain drowsy or 'post-ictal' for some time. They should be observed carefully and kept in the recovery position until they are able to maintain their own airway. If it is the child's first convulsion the parents will require much reassurance and will need to be taught how to manage future episodes. This will include prescribing buccal midazolam or rectal diazepam to be administered at home.

Status epilepticus

Seizures may be very prolonged and are an important cause of coma. Status epilepticus is defined as continuous seizure activity for more than 30 minutes or a series of seizures without full recovery in between. Status may occur following febrile convulsions or more commonly in children with known epilepsy, or with other acute causes such as trauma or metabolic disturbance. The child's airway should be opened, oxygen given and blood glucose checked. Anticonvulsant medication should be given as described below. (*I assumes treatment box is below!*) Any child with very prolonged seizures should be monitored carefully on an intensive care unit, and urgent investigations performed to identify the cause.

KEY POINTS

- Febrile convulsions occur in 3% of children between age 5 months and 5 years. The prognosis is usually excellent.
- Children who are fitting must be placed in the recovery position and their airway maintained.
- Always check blood sugar as hypoglycaemia is a common and treatable cause.
- Any convulsion lasting more than 10 minutes should be terminated with buccal midazolam or rectal diazepam.
- Status epilepticus is fitting for more than 30 minutes and requires urgent treatment.

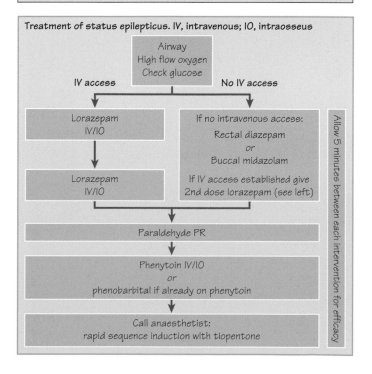

Treatment of status epilepticus. IV, intravenous; IO, intraosseus

Accidents

Each year in the UK about 300 children are killed and 10,000 permanently injured by accidents. About 2 million children a year attend hospitals each year due to accidents. Nearly half of these have occurred in the home. Most accidents are not just chance events but are to some extent predictable, and therefore preventable. As most accidents occur in and around the home, one of the main accident-prevention strategies is parental education and improving the awareness of potential hazards. Some of the common causes of accidents and their prevention strategies are listed below.

Choking
• Keep small toys away from toddlers
• No nuts for children under 5 years
• Use pens with safe tops

▶ **Road traffic accidents**
This is the most common cause of accidental death in childhood. The child is usually a pedestrian or cyclist. Road traffic accidents can be prevented by reducing the speed of traffic and by educating both drivers and children
• Use child car seats and seatbelts
• Teach road safety to children from a young age
• Traffic calming schemes around schools and playgrounds
• Cycle helmets reduce the number of serious head injuries in cyclists
• Enforce speed limits by use of speed cameras
• Improve access to specialized trauma and neurosurgical centres

Drowning
• Mostly occurs in fresh water (baths, swimming pools, rivers)
• Outcome is better in very cold water due to protective effect of hypothermia
• If the child is resuscitated from a near-drowning, the outcome is usually good
Prevention
• Never leave children unattended in the bath
• Swim only where a lifeguard is present
• Fence off pools and ponds

Falls
• Fit stair gates at home
• Fit child-proof window locks
• Soft surfaces in playgrounds

Poisoning (See Chapter 60)

Burns

Every year 37 000 children attend hospital Emergency Departments with burns or scalds. Burns are the second most common cause of accidental death in childhood after road traffic accidents, and account for about 90 deaths a year. Fatal burns are usually associated with house fires. Half are due to smoke inhalation and half to direct burns. Death from burns arises due to the massive fluid loss through the exposed tissues and due to infection. The severity of a burn is determined by the temperature and the duration of contact. Most skin burns are due to scalding with hot water or hot drinks

Prevention
• Caution in the kitchen
• Reduce hot water temperature to 48°C
• Install smoke detectors
• Avoid trailing flexes on kettles and irons
• Use fire guards
• Cover electrical sockets

4%
40%
4%
7%
7%

Trunk represents
20% back
20% front

Management
Remove the heat source and any hot clothing immediately. Cool the skin under a cold tap and wrap the area in a clean sheet or cover with clean clingfilm. If there has been smoke inhalation check for wheeze, cyanosis or respiratory distress. There may be soot in the nose and mouth. Check oxygen saturation and carboxy-haemoglobin level (in case of carbon monoxide poisoning). Give high flow oxygen and consider ventilation. The extent of the burns should be assessed and the percentage of the body surface area affecting full-thickness or partial thickness burns should be estimated (palms of hand = 1%). Burns affecting >10% are highly significant and intravenous fluid resuscitation will be required. The fluid management is complicated and depends on the percentage area affected. Give morphine to control pain. Full-thickness burns are less painful than partial ones. Most burns victims are now treated in specialized burns units. Skin grafting may be necessary and psychological support will be needed for the child and the family, especially if there is extensive scarring

Accidental ingestion in young children

Accidental poisoning is becoming less common as parents become more aware of the risks and drugs are sold in child-resistant containers. Accidental poisoning most commonly occurs in inquisitive toddlers, especially when they are staying in grandparents' homes where there are likely to be more medicines and household products may be stored less carefully

Common drugs ingested
- Aspirin
- Paracetamol
- Antidepressants

Common household agents
- Disinfectants
- Bleach
- Weedkiller
- Paraffin or white spirit
- Dishwasher tablets

History and evaluation
- Substance ingested
- Time ingested
- Calculate maximum quantity that may have been ingested
- Inspect the product container

Examination
- What is the child's conscious level and are the pupils reacting normally?
- Check pulse and blood pressure and monitor if arrhythmias are likely
- Is there evidence in the mouth of ingestion, e.g. ulcers, or clues from the clothing, such as burns or smell?

Investigations
- Blood and urine for toxicology if the poison is not known
- Paracetamol, alcohol, salicylate or drug levels, as appropriate
- Blood glucose, especially in alcohol poisoning
- Keep the product and packaging for further analysis

Management
- Discuss with nearest poisons unit
- Where possible remove the poison. Gastric lavage should not be used routinely but may be considered if a life-threatening quantity of a drug (e.g. aspirin) has been ingested within the last hour. Lavage is contraindicated if the airway cannot be protected
- Activated charcoal can absorb many drugs (e.g. aspirin, paracetamol, phenytoin, carbamazepine) but should only be given if a life-threatening quantity has been ingested within the last hour. Multiple dose charcoal therapy may be helpful in some situations
- Inducing vomiting with ipecacuanha syrup is dangerous and no longer recommended
- Give specific antidote if available (e.g. naloxone for opiates, vitamin K for warfarin)
- Supportive treatment for respiration. Monitor for cardiac arrhythmias and treat as necessary
- Advice should be given to parents on safety within the home

Intentional overdose in older children and adolescents

Agents used to overdose
- ▶ Paracetamol
- Aspirin
- Alcohol
- Drugs of abuse (e.g. opiates)
- ▶ Sedatives and antidepressants

Risk factors for overdose
- Children in care
- Emotional upset
- Child abuse or bullying
- Psychiatric illness
- Suicidal thoughts (usually rare)
- Other self-harming behaviour

Paracetamol poisoning
- Rarely severe enough to cause serious problems but liver failure can occur after ingestion of 20–30 tablets and is likely if >150 mg/kg of paracetamol has been ingested
- If >150 mg/kg ingested start treatment immediately with IV N-acetlycysteine and oral methionine. These must be commenced within 8 h of ingestion. These antidotes can be stopped if the serum concentration falls below the treatment line
- Serum paracetamol levels should be measured 4 h after ingestion and the level plotted on a nomogram. If above the treatment level, an infusion of N-acetyl cysteine should be commenced and continued for at least 24 h. This reduces the risk of liver damage
- In significant overdoses, serial measurements of liver enzymes and coagulation times should be made to monitor hepatic function. Serum urea and electrolytes should be used to monitor renal function
- The initial symptoms of nausea and vomiting usually settle within 24 h but hepatic necrosis can occur 3–4 days later with the onset of right upper quadrant pain and later encephalopathy
- In the most severe cases (acidosis, encephalopathy or severe coagulopathy) urgent liver transplantation may be life-saving

Management
- Evaluation, history and examination, as above
- Removal of poison where possible or administration of charcoal
- Aspirin remains in the stomach for a considerable time and gastric lavage should be considered
- Treatment of the toxic effects of drug, as above
- Admission for assessment by child psychiatrist in all cases
- Consider the possibility of serious risk factors, such as abuse

Living with a chronic condition

More common chronic conditions in childhood
- Asthma (moderate and severe)
- Epilepsy
- Congenital heart disease
- Diabetes mellitus
- Arthritis
- Cystic fibrosis
- Chronic renal failure
- Malignancy

Factors affecting a child's adjustment to a chronic illness

The child
- The age of the child
- The age at which the illness developed. School entry and adolescence are particularly vulnerable periods
- Low intelligence or unattractiveness increase the probability of maladjustment

The illness
- Conditions with unpredictable flare-ups or recurrences are more stressful than stable conditions
- 'Invisible' conditions (e.g. diabetes) may be concealed and lead to a lack of acceptance

The family
- The family's attitude and ability to function is the most critical factor in determining the child's adjustment
- Positive warm family relationships support children
- The family need to be interested and engaged in managing the illness, attending clinics, complying with treatment and seeking help when problems occur

OUT PATIENTS

What you need from your evaluation

Assessment
- What is the extent of the disease and its complications in the child?
- What are the physical effects (e.g. poor growth, delayed puberty) of the illness on the child?
- How has the illness affected the child's performance at home, at school and with peers?
- What is the level of school absence?
- How has the child adjusted to the illness?
- What impact does the child's illness have on the family and its members?
- Does the child understand their illness and take responsibility for their management?
- How has the family adjusted to the special impact or burden of the illness?
- Who is acting as main carer? What support do they get?
- Has there been change in parents work or relationship?
- Have siblings had any emotional or behavioural difficulties?

Management
- Try to confine the consequences of the condition to the minimum manifestation
- Encourage normal growth and development
- Assist the child in maximizing their potential in all possible areas
- Prevent or diminish the behavioural and social consequences of a chronic condition

A chronic medical condition is defined as *an illness that lasts longer than 3 months, and is sufficiently severe to interfere with a child's ordinary activities*. According to the UK General Household Survey, as many as 10–20% of children experience a longstanding medical condition, with 5–10% having a moderately to severe long-term illness or disability.

The effect of chronic illness on the child

It is not only the severity and prognosis of a condition that influences how a child adjusts. In fact there appears to be little relationship between the severity of the condition and the extent of psychosocial difficulties. Children with mild disabilities may suffer as much or more than those where the condition is severe.

It is perhaps not so surprising that emotional, behavioural and educational difficulties are two to three times more likely than in healthy children. Low self-esteem, impaired self-image, behavioural problems, depression, anxiety and school dysfunction are all common. They may result from the child's own response to the chronic illness or relate to how parents, peers, professionals and society react.

Children's ability to perform at school can be affected, placing them at risk for becoming underachievers and failures in their own eyes and the eyes of their peers. School is often missed because of acute exacerbations, outpatient appointments and hospitalizations. Chronic illness affects social aspects of school life too. Frequent illness episodes and restrictions may exclude children from activities. Physical appearance, acute medical problems, taking medications at school and special diets all can contribute.

The effect of chronic illness on the family

When parents learn that their child has a chronic illness they tend to respond in a way similar to experiencing a bereavement. The initial reaction is shock or disbelief, followed by denial, anger and resentment, and eventually reaching an acceptance of the situation. It is not surprising that clinical anxiety, depression, guilt and grief are common, particularly for mothers, who often take the major caring role. It is also not surprising that marital problems may be exacerbated.

Siblings may also be at higher risk. Anxiety, embarrassment, resentment and guilt are common, as are fears about their own well-being and the cause and nature of their sibling's health problems. Parents may be less available to their healthy children, and they may also neglect, overindulge or develop unrealistic expectations for them.

We tend to focus on psychopathology and psychosocial problems when considering chronic illness, but it is important to remember that the impact is not always negative. Some families seem to grow closer to each other and provide outstanding care for their children. The question often arises: 'How do some families of chronically ill children survive so well?'

The paediatric care of children with long-term medical conditions

Paediatric care of children with chronic illnesses needs to be holistic and go beyond clinical management alone. Time, good communication and skill are needed. This is particularly so around the time of diagnosis, and also at transition points such as starting school or during adolescence. At times, parents may need the opportunity to talk without their child being present, and adolescents should also be encouraged to be seen on their own—to talk about problems, and also to begin to be responsible for their own health care. The role of the paediatrician includes:

- **Counselling:** Concern and empathy can go a long way in assisting the family to make the best of the circumstances they face. It is important that the family knows that concealing a chronic condition (where that is possible) is rarely helpful as it encourages the child to believe that the illness is a secret and something shameful.
- **Education:** An important aspect of management is educating the family about the condition. This increases trust and provides the family with skills to self-manage many aspects of the condition—particularly critical in conditions such as asthma and diabetes.
- **Coordination:** Children with chronic conditions are often looked after by a variety of health professionals: consultants, therapists and dietitians, not to mention teachers and social workers. Liaison and coordination are very important as differing opinions and advice can be very confusing for the family. Specialist clinics can be helpful, especially when there is a specialist nurse to take on this role as well as offer close support.
- **Genetic issues:** Parents often have questions about genetic implications for other children, and the affected child's own chances of fertility. A genetics referral may be appropriate.
- **Support:** Chronic illness can be an isolating experience and many families do not have the support of extended family and friends. A referral to social services may be needed for advice about benefits and other services. If there are emotional and behavioural difficulties, referral for counselling may also be required. Self-help and voluntary organizations such as Diabetes UK or Epilepsy Action can be helpful and often run support groups and activities allowing families with similar problems to meet.

Involvement with school

Good liaison with school is important. Staff need to understand about the medical condition so that they can cope competently with problems. Their greatest concern is usually around acute exacerbations, but they may also need to dispense medication or understand dietary restrictions. Asking teachers to report untoward events such as symptoms or drug side-effects can be helpful. A formal health care plan should be prepared to give instructions on the illness, emergency procedures and key contact details.

A child who is underachieving needs extra support. This may include help in making up work lost through absence or providing preferential seating in class. Teachers can be instrumental in helping children cope and integrate socially into school life—particularly important if the family is not coping well. Some children may have special educational requirements that need to be met (Chapter 63).

KEY POINTS

- Chronic and recurrent medical problems are not uncommon
- They have a broad impact on both the child and the family
- A holistic approach involving the whole family is important
- Paediatric care should involve support, coordination of care and liaison with other professionals and school

Prevalence of disability

8 per 10,000 children have a significant disability of which the most common are:
- **Physical and multiple disabilities**
  Cerebral palsy
  Muscular dystrophy
  Spinal disorders
- **Severe learning difficulties**
  Chromosomal abnormalities
  CNS abnormality
  Idiopathic
  Autism
- **Special senses**
  Severe visual handicap
  Severe hearing loss

How disability presents

- Antenatally or at birth if anomalies are present
- In the first year for motor handicaps and severe learning disabilities
- In the second or third year for moderate learning disabilities, language disorder and autism
- After cranial insults

Assessment of disability

This involves:
- A detailed assessment of the child's abilities
- Recognition of any underlying medical problem
- An assessment of the likely long-term difficulties

A Child Development Team is involved for complex difficulties	
Professional	Role
Developmental paediatrician	Diagnosis of medical problems. Advice on medical issues
Physiotherapist	Assessment and management of gross motor difficulties, abnormal tone and prevention of deformities in cerebral palsy. Provision of special equipment
Occupational therapist	Assessment and management of fine motor difficulties. Advice on toys, play and appliances to aid daily living
Speech and language therapist	Advice on feeding. Assessment and management of speech, language and all aspects of communication
Psychologist	Support and counselling of family and team
Special needs teacher	Advice on special educational needs
Social worker	Support for the family. Advice on social service benefits, respite care, etc.
Liaison health visitor	Support for the family. Liaison with local health visitor

Management of disability

- **Giving the diagnosis:** this must be carried out in a skilled way by a senior professional
- **Medical management:** therapists' input should be provided initially at home or the child development centre, and then in nursery and school
- **Genetic counselling:** required by many families even if no obvious genetic cause is identified
- **Education:** A Statement of Special Educational Needs describes the educational provision that must be made for a child with disabilities. Where possible the child should be integrated into mainstream school
- **Provision of services:** Social Services are responsible for preschool childcare, respite care, home help, advice about benefits and assessment for services on leaving school. Voluntary agencies may provide support and information

Living with a disability

- Parents' initial reaction to news of their child's disability is similar to bereavement; they may feel shock, fear and loss, anger and guilt. Each stage of childhood then requires further adaptation, and independence is an ongoing issue
- Schools need to be prepared for any anticipated difficulties and to accommodate physical disabilities. Staff must work with therapists to implement their recommendations. Young adult disability teams can advise about options beyond high school

Children with disabilities have complex health needs. Many of the issues described in Chapter 61 are relevant to families with a disabled child. It is important to appreciate the terminology relating to disability.

A *disorder* is a medically definable condition or disease; an *impairment* is a loss of function; *disability* refers to any restriction of ability (resulting from an impairment) and *handicap* is the impact of the impairment on the child's activities.

The distinction between disability and handicap is important. One of the aims is to minimize the handicap that results from disability. It is important to consider how people with disability are perceived by society—there are ongoing issues of poor accessibility, prejudice and discrimination affecting people with disability.

Some parents will describe their child as having 'special needs' rather than as either disabled or handicapped. This term is used by professionals in discussion with families and in the educational setting when a child may have a *Statement of Special Educational Needs*.

How disability presents

Children with disabilities may be identified as a result of parental or professional concern. A syndrome or central nervous system abnormality may be identified in the antenatal period or at birth. Babies with neonatal problems are followed up closely as they are at high risk of disability. Deafness, motor handicaps and severe learning disabilities often become apparent during the first year. Moderate or even severe learning disabilities, language disorder and autism may not be recognized until the child is 2 or 3 years of age, when it becomes clear that their developmental progress is not normal. Problems may arise in later childhood after acute illness events such as head injury or brain tumour.

Assessment and diagnosis of a child with a disability

Identifying the underlying medical problem is one aspect of the assessment. There is also a developmental evaluation and an assessment of how the difficulties are likely to impact on the child's family and school life. When difficulties are complex, a Child Development Team should be involved (see adjacent box).

Paediatric care

A holistic approach is needed. Sensitive support is important while parents come to terms with their child's difficulties and at each transition. Care often involves a number of professionals, both medical and non-medical, from different specialties and agencies. It can be helpful for families to have a named professional who acts as their key worker in coordinating the multidisciplinary team, e.g. arranging outpatient visits to different therapists on the same day to reduce absence from school.

The diagnosis of a disability is usually devastating and the way that the diagnosis is communicated is important, coming at the start of a long doctor–patient relationship. The session should be conducted in private by a senior doctor with both parents present. There should be opportunity for questions, with a follow-up session arranged shortly after. If a baby is born with congenital anomalies, consultation with parents should take place as concerns arise, with the baby present, sharing with the family the concerns and describing the process of making a definitive diagnosis.

Once the child's difficulties have been fully assessed, developmental therapy is required. This may be delivered in the child development centre, at home or at nursery. Once the child is in full-time school, the services are often delivered by community therapists who work with the child and advise school staff.

Provision of services

Agencies other than health are involved in providing services to the family:
• **Education services** are responsible for assessing learning difficulties, providing preschool home teaching, nursery schooling and education both in mainstream and special schools. Children who require medical treatments in school (such as drugs via gastros-

tomy) should have a written health care plan agreed to support staff in giving the child's treatment
• **Social services** are responsible for providing preschool child care, relief care, advice about benefits and assessment for services needed on leaving school. Child protection concerns also fall into their area.
• **Voluntary organizations** provide support and information for families, run play facilities, provide educational opportunities and sitting services. Some are large national agencies with numerous local branches, others are smaller groups concerned with a local issue or a single diagnosis.

The child with special educational needs

Children with special needs are educated in mainstream schools where possible. Extra help with learning and physical difficulties is provided in the classroom. This often involves a special needs assistant for the child, and may also include physiotherapy, occupational therapy and speech and language therapy. Mainstream placement has the advantage of integrating children with special needs into a local peer group and encourages their inclusion in society from an early age. It has the benefit that other children learn to live alongside children with disabilities and view this as normal. However, there can be disadvantages such as large classes, less specific support and buildings poorly adapted for physical difficulties.

Special schools provide teaching in smaller classes. Staff have a greater experience of complex medical needs. The disadvantage is that children are not included in a wider social group. An alternative approach is to have specialist units within a mainstream setting.

The Statement of Special Educational Needs

The education authority is obliged to assess children who need additional provision because of severe or complex difficulties. The assessment includes reports from an educational psychologist, a paediatrician and other professionals such as therapists and the child's nursery or school. It clarifies the medical needs, the educational needs, the needs for physical assistance, supervision and transport. A legally binding document is produced called the Statement of Special Educational Needs. The child's educational needs and the necessary support are stated and these are reviewed on an annual basis.

Transition to adult services

There is a statutory requirement that social services make a formal assessment of a child's long-term needs as they approach adult years for those children with a Statement of Special Educational Needs with complex health or disability problems. The assessment is conducted with information from health, education services, the young person and family. Transition from the long-term paediatric medical team, therapists and education setting to adult health and social care is difficult and needs careful planning. Children with severe complex needs may need residential care as adults or significant extra support to live independently. There is a need for ongoing support from specialist clinicians with expertise in adult learning disability.

Prevalence
- 4 per 1000 children

Aetiology/pathophysiology
- Chromosome disorders — 30%
- Identifiable disorders or syndromes — 20%
- Associated with cerebral palsy, microcephaly, infantile spasms, postnatal cerebral insults — 20%
- Metabolic or degenerative disease — <1%
- Idiopathic — 25%

Clinical features
- Reduced intellectual functioning
- Delay in reaching developmental milestones, particularly language and social skills, in early childhood
- Often associated with:
  Epilepsy
  Vision and hearing deficits
  Communication problems
  Attention deficit/hyperactivity
  Feeding problems and failure to thrive
  Microcephaly

How learning disability presents
- Dysmorphic features may be noted at birth
- SLD presents as developmental delay before 12 months
- MLD often presents with delayed language in toddlers
- The diagnostic process is discussed in Chapter 3

Management (needs to be multidisciplinary)
- Attempt to find underlying cause
- Early intervention and educational programmes to stimulate cognitive, language and motor development
- Attention to special educational needs, with Statement if severe
- Behavioural difficulties must be addressed
- Family support and benefits should be provided
- General paediatric care must not be neglected

Paediatric follow-up
- Developmental progress and physical growth require review
- Screening for specific associated problems in some conditions
- Behaviour is often an issue
- Liaison with other professionals is important, particularly regarding education
- The family needs support

Prognosis
- Depends on the underlying cause
- Degree of independent living relates to the severity of learning disability and the underlying aetiology

Children are said to have a learning disability when they experience significantly greater difficulty than their peers in making progress with intellectual developmental skills. Intellect overlaps with all other developmental areas, so severe learning difficulty is normally part of a pattern of global developmental delay linked with problems of mobility, communication and self-care skills.

There can be many reasons why a child may have learning difficulties. There may be a clear pathological cause such as Down's syndrome or brain injury. Learning difficulties may arise as a result of neglect in early life. In many cases there is no clear genetic, neuroanatomical, metabolic or environmental cause that can be identified. This is an evolving area of medicine and ongoing advances in genetics and brain imaging science help understand a greater proportion of these problems.

Learning disability is termed mild, moderate, severe or profound according to the intellectual limitation and degree of independent self-care. Children and adults with *profound* learning disability are totally dependent on their carers for all activities of daily living including self-care and feeding, and usually have very limited communication. Those with *severe* learning difficulties may learn limited self-care and simple communication skills, but will not be able to live independently. Those with *mild* or *moderate* learning disability may live independently with support.

Paediatric management
The role of the paediatrician is to assess patterns of early development that may indicate a significant future developmental problem, to diagnose the underlying cause through examination and

investigation, communicate openly with the family to ensure there is understanding of the problems and the likely future implications, to manage medical problems and to coordinate multidisciplinary developmental therapy and multiagency liaison for the child.

Growing up with learning disability

The diagnosis of severe learning disability is devastating and families require particularly sensitive support at diagnosis and beyond. Each stage of childhood brings its own issues from starting school to adulthood. Adolescence is usually a particularly difficult time when issues related to independent living, friendships and sexuality, vocational training and care into later adult years may arise. Transition away from the well-known childrens' services to adult services also presents difficulties and needs planning with social care staff.

It is important to begin therapeutic input early to stimulate cognitive, language and motor development. Therapists from the Child Development Team provide advice on play activities to stimulate development and maximize function. Parents learn about methods of communication with speech therapy and alternative communication systems such as Makaton signing or visual language cards if necessary. Attendance at specialist preschool nursery can be enjoyable and promote social learning for the child. This also gives parents contact with other families.

Many children with learning disabilities are included in mainstream nursery and primary school, with appropriate help provided. Others, particularly if they have additional disabilities, may be better placed in a specialist school. Depending on the degree of disability, a Statement of Special Educational Needs may be needed (see Chapter 62). Education goals must be realistic, and should include skills such as personal care, development of social behaviour, and independence. On leaving school, facilities should be available for the young adult which may include specialist accommodation and further vocational education placement.

Behavioural problems occur with greater frequency in children with developmental disabilities. This may include attention difficulties, hyperactivity (see Chapter 12), stereotypic or self-injury behaviour. Psychological help is often needed to understand difficult behaviours and advise on strategies for management. Medical problems such as eyesight, hearing, gastrointestinal symptoms, nutrition issues, seizures and acute illness need active management.

It is difficult for health staff to assess children with learning disability when acute illness occurs. A problem such as acute appendicitis can be very difficult to detect in a patient with no speech communication and limited understanding. Health staff need training in the specialist needs of people with learning disability to provide good care.

Down's syndrome (trisomy 21)

Down's syndrome is an example of a condition which causes significant learning disability with implications for long-term independent living. Down's syndrome is the commonest genetic anomaly causing learning disability. The extra chromosome is usually maternal, and the incidence of Down's syndrome increases with maternal age (1% at age 40 years).

Features include facial features of upward sloping palpebral fissures, folds of skin over the epicanthus of the eyes, a protruding tongue, flat occiput, single palmar creases, and mild to moderate developmental delay. Associated medical problems include gas-

trointestinal problems (most commonly duodenal atresia), 40–50% have cardiac anomalies (most commonly atrioventricular canal defects), otitis media, squint, hypothyroidism, atlanto-axial vertebral instability and leukaemia.

Fragile X

Fragile X is an important genetic cause of learning disabilities among boys. The diagnosis should be sought in any boy who has unexplained moderate or severe learning disability. Some girls carrying the chromosome have mild learning disabilities.

Autistic spectrum disorders

Autism is a developmental disorder with abnormal behaviours in three key elements:
• Poor verbal and non-verbal communication (often reduced eye contact)
• Obsessive intense repetitive interests
• Reduced imaginative play.

Autism is sometimes described as a 'mind-blindness'—an inability to relate to others, to understand that someone else might view something in a different way. There is evidence of genetic factors in a number of children with autism.

There is a broad spectrum of severity of autism. In severe autism language development is profoundly impaired and behaviours are often extremely difficult to manage. There are a number of children with some, but not all, features of the autistic spectrum. An example is *Asperger's syndrome* in which language development is usually good but social empathy is poor, leading to problems with peer relationships and school progress.

Specialist education support is required and the family need support to manage difficult behaviours and communication at home and school.

KEY POINTS

• Where possible, the underlying condition should be diagnosed.
• The child's developmental progress should be monitored.
• Appropriate input should be provided in the preschool years and appropriate school placement made.
• The child and parents need a supportive framework.
• Transition to adult services needs careful planning.

Visual impairment

A child is partially sighted if visual acuity is less than 6/18 and therefore educational aids such as large print books can be used. A child is defined as blind if visual acuity is <3/60 and therefore education can only be provided by methods such as Braille that do not involve sight.

Prevalence

1 in 2500 children are registered blind or partially sighted and 50% have additional functional impairments.

Aetiology

The commonest causes are optic atrophy, congenital cataracts and choroidoretinal degeneration.

Clinical features

The eyes of visually impaired children may look abnormal or there may be unusual movements. When children are visually impaired from birth, their psychomotor development is altered. Early smiling is inconsistent and they do not turn towards sound. Reaching out for objects and the development of a pincer grip is delayed. Although early language may be normal, the development of more complex language may be slower. 'Blindisms' (eye poking, eye rubbing and rocking) may occur. Hearing deficit or severe learning difficulties are commonly associated problems.

How visual impairment presents

In neonates the diagnosis is suspected if cataracts, nystagmus or purposeless eye movements are present. Otherwise it may be identified by parents or through child health surveillance. If there is any suspicion of visual impairment, an ophthalmological examination is required which may involve visual evoked response (VER) testing.

Management

Early intervention needs to focus on developmental progress, reducing blindisms and increasing parental confidence. Expert teaching assistance for educational support is needed to advise on approach to learning, mobility and support services.

Growing up with visual impairment

Parents need advice on how to care for their child, adaptations for the home and how to provide stimulation in a non-visual way. Mainstream preschool is usually appropriate with support. Beyond this, placement depends on learning abilities and may be at mainstream school, a partially sighted unit or school for the blind. Mobility training is an important aspect of education.

Hearing impairment

Prevalence

Four per cent of children have hearing deficits. Most are mild but 2 per 1000 need a hearing aid and 1 per 1000 needs special education.

Aetiology

Most mild to moderate hearing loss is conductive, and is secondary to otitis media. Sensorineural deafness may be genetic, may result from pre- or perinatal problems or follow a cerebral insult.

Factors that increase the risk of deafness

Neurosensory	Conductive
History of meningitis	Cleft palate
Cerebral palsy	Recurrent otitis media
Family history of deafness	
Aminoglycoside treatment	
Congenital cytomegalovirus infection	

How hearing impairment presents

Universal neonatal screening with otoautistic emissions (OAE) is now being introduced to identify congenital sensorineural loss. Audiological testing should be requested for children at risk (see above), any child with significantly delayed or unclear speech or where there is parental suspicion of deafness. Investigations may include brainstem evoked responses (BSER) if the child is young or unable to cooperate.

Clinical features

Hearing impairment may manifest itself in a number of ways:
- A lack of response to sound
- Delayed speech
- Behavioural problems
- Associated problems: learning disabilities, neurological disorders, visual deficits.

Management

Grommets are inserted in children with persistent conductive hearing loss. Hearing aids are fitted for sensorineural deafness, and early speech therapy is needed to develop communication. Cochlear implant surgery may be considered for moderate to severe sensorineural deafness. Genetic counselling may be needed.

Growing up with hearing impairment

Parents need to learn to communicate with the child, which may include sign language. Moderately deaf children can attend mainstream school. Severely deaf children require specialist education in a hearing unit attached to a mainstream school, or at a special school for the deaf. Deaf children have a higher risk of psychological developmental disorders.

Types of abuse and neglect

Emotional abuse
- 'Frozen, watchful' appearance
- Expressionless face, wary eyes
- Abnormally affectionate to strangers

Non-accidental injury
- Bruises of suspicious shape or site
- Burns and scalds
- Bites
- Hidden head injuries
- Suspicious fractures

Sexual abuse
- Anogenital bruising and tears if acute
- Pregnancy, sexually transmitted diseases
- There may be no physical signs

Physical neglect
- Unkempt dirty appearance
- Sores
- Uncared-for nappy rash
- Failure to thrive

What you need from your evaluation

History

- **How was the injury incurred?** Characteristically, the explanation is unconvincing, does not match the injury and there is a delay on obtaining medical advice. It is particularly suspicious if young not-yet-mobile infants have been injured
- **Past medical history.** Ask about previous injuries
- **Development and behaviour.** Both are affected by neglect and abuse
- **Social history and family history.** Find out who is in the home and who cares for the child. Abuse is more likely where there are changes in partner. Other professionals (e.g. health visitors and nursery nurses) can often provide extra details

Investigations and their significance

As the implications of non-accidental injury are so serious, rare medical causes of excessive bruising or fragile bones must be ruled out

● Photographs	Useful for further consultation and evidence in court
● Full blood count, bleeding time, PT and PTT	To rule out haematological causes of excessive bruising
● Skeletal survey (radiographs)	Certain fractures (of ribs, spiral fractures and metaphyseal chips in the long bones) and fractures at various stages of healing are particularly suspicious
● Pregnancy test and cultures (in sexual abuse)	The finding of sexually transmitted disease is strong corroborative evidence (and requires treatment)

Physical examination

- **General appearance.** Are there signs of neglect? Is the child particularly wary or over-affectionate towards the examiner?
- **Growth.** Plot measurements and weight and compare with previous measurements. Abused and neglected children often fail to thrive
- **Injuries.** Many non-accidental injuries have a characteristic appearance. Multiple injuries are suspicious, particularly if sustained at different times
  - **Bruises:** Bruises, except on toddlers' legs, may be suspicious. The pattern may indicate how they were acquired. The age (identified from colour) may help in refuting an implausible explanation
  - **Burns and scalds:** Inflicted scalds are classically symmetrical without splash marks. Inflicted cigarette burns cause deep circular ulcers
  - **Bites:** The dental impression can be used forensically to identify the perpetrator
  - **Bony injuries:** Clinical evidence of fractures may be found
- **Neurological examination.** Retinal haemorrhages are a clue to subdural haemorrhage, which can occur when a baby is shaken
- **Signs of sexual abuse.** If sexual abuse is suspected, the genitalia and anus must be examined by an experienced paediatrician. Signs may be overt, such as bruising and tears, or subtle. The absence of signs does not refute the diagnosis

Overview

Children are dependent on their carers for their physical, emotional and developmental needs, their supervision and safety. It is hard to understand that adults can harm children—yet this occurs commonly. Abuse is typically carried out by family members or friends who have close contact with children. Health professionals need to understand the different presentations of child abuse and how to work with agencies to safeguard children.

How does child abuse present?

Child abuse can present in many ways. Some of the more common scenarios are:

• A parent or teacher seeks help following an episode of abuse which the child has disclosed.
• Families present a child to primary care or the emergency department with non-specific signs of illness or injury. Evaluation reveals inconsistencies in the history, background social risk factors or physical signs which indicate abuse.
• Physical signs of abuse are detected during routine contacts.
• Abused children may have emotional or behavioural problems such as poor mood, anxiety, poor social interaction, attention problems, aggressive behaviours, sexualized behaviours.

Physical abuse

Physical injuries are usually inflicted when adults lose emotional control while caring for babies and children. Risk factors include parental stress, substance abuse, poor social support, and situations where parents have suffered abusive experience in their own childhood. Injuries can occur with premeditation such as deliberate physical punishment. Injuries may range in severity from minor bruises to fatal brain or abdominal injury. Injuries may recur over an extended period of time, through years of childhood. A child who has suffered a minor abusive injury is at risk of a future severe injury.

Any type of injury may have an abusive cause and there may be many different mechanisms including; punching, slapping, kicking, biting, hitting with an object, abdominal trauma, fractures, shaking, burns, scalds, asphyxiation, poisoning.

Factors that indicate abusive injury include:

• Carer conceals injury
• Delay in presentation for medical assessment of injury
• Unusual or inconsistent history of mechanism of injury
• Multiple injuries
• Different age injuries
• Some specific injuries are typical of abuse
• Previous social concerns
• Child discloses abusive injury.

Some injury patterns are more highly suggestive of abuse:

• **Bruises**: distinctive shapes such as bite marks, multiple bruises in young babies, unusual sites on the body
• **Burns**: cigarette burn, immersion hot water scald injuries
• **Fractures**: young babies, multiple fractures, different age fractures
• **Shaken baby pattern**: subdural haematoma brain injury with retinal haemorrhages and skeletal fractures.

Neglect

Neglect is inadequate care which can result in serious harm to a child. Basic care is to provide food, warmth, clothing, hygiene, dental care and immunizations, and to seek medical attention for an illness. Parents should act to protect children from harm by injury. Basic care involves good parenting behaviours including establishing boundaries relating to children's behaviour and a healthy lifestyle of diet, exercise, activity.

Neglect and failure to thrive

Some young children fail to thrive with poor nutrition. Good infant feeding requires a good emotional interaction during the feed. Parents need to be responsive to the child, manage periods of difficulty, seek advice if there are problems. This can be impaired if parents have poor models of parenting, social stresses, mental health problems or substance abuse problems.

Children can present with problems of faltering growth, acute illness and developmental problems. If admitted to hospital these babies often show rapid weight gain. Catch-up growth may occur but brain development may be disrupted. Subsequent emotional and educational problems are common.

Emotional abuse

Attachment is the close emotional bond which binds families—the relationships in which children learn skills for future relationships and independence. Quality of attachment depends on quality and consistency of parent–child interaction.

Children suffer emotional abuse if exposed to persistent or severe ill-treatment with dysfunctional parental responses such as rejection, excessive punishment, isolation, scapegoating, manipulation or overprotection. Emotional abuse also includes giving children inappropriate responsibilities and allowing children to witness harmful adult actions such as domestic violence.

The consequences of emotional abuse are profound. Children fail to learn normal emotional responses. They may develop problems in empathy, self-esteem, resilience and independence. There is usually significant emotional abuse in all forms of physical abuse, sexual abuse and neglect.

Sexual abuse

Sexual abuse is inappropriate sexual behaviour involving a child such as exposing a child to pornography, sexual touching, involvement in sexual acts, vaginal, oral or rectal intercourse. Perpetrators are most commonly family members or acquaintances. Perpetrators befriend ('groom') children to create situations of close contact. Perpetrators use threats to discourage children from disclosing abuse and may give children drugs or alcohol.

Sexual abuse is disclosed if a child talks about what has happened. An abused child may demonstrate inappropriate sexual language or behaviour in their play. Abuse may be suspected from a pattern of soft tissue trauma (mouth, anus or genitalia) or infection. Abuse can cause non-specific illness symptoms or behavioural problems. If children feel safe they may be able to tell a trusted adult relative or teacher that someone has hurt them. Staff need to be able to talk to children in a way that lets them disclose what has happened through open and supportive questions.

Sensitive, skilled medical management is required. General examination and anogenital examination with a colposcope is performed to document injuries and obtain photographic and forensic evidence. Following sexual abuse, physical signs are commonly absent.

Victims of abuse need future safeguarding and follow-up psychological support to address the emotional harm of the abuse.

Factitious or fabricated illness

There are situations where adults present children for medical investigation with illness symptoms or signs that have been fabricated. This can lead to extensive medical investigation which can physically and emotionally harm the child. There are complex reasons for these behaviours—possibly a form of inappropriate care-seeking behaviour which may reflect a background personality disorder.

Medical investigation

A full skeletal survey radiography series is performed in infants where there is concern about previous physical abuse. Brain imaging and ophthalmology review are performed to investigate for shaking injury.

From the medical assessment, it is usually possible to differentiate between abusive injuries and rare disorders that predispose to fractures or brain injury.

Blood tests to exclude haematological problem such as coagulation or platelet disorder may be performed in children with bruising injuries.

Screening for sexually transmitted infection, pregnancy and forensic testing may be performed following sexual abuse.

The safeguarding process

Professionals must report incidents that raise concern to the statutory authority with responsibility for child welfare. In the UK it is the local authority social services department that will investigate a situation of concern. It is best practice to keep families informed at all stages of the process and communicate clearly why actions are being taken.

Medical assessment is part of the investigation of a concern. Careful documentation of the history (including the child's own words), examination and medical investigation is essential. The paediatrician gives an opinion on the features in the history and examination findings. Background information is shared with other professionals such as health visitors, nursery nurses, social workers, the GP and school. This gives a picture of the risk factors in the family and any previous concerns. A multi-agency case conference meeting is held to review the combined assessments, decide the level of risk and agree how to protect the child.

If a child is at risk then a safeguarding plan is put in place with key professionals to work with the family and monitor the future welfare of the child. In many situations it is possible for the child to remain in the care of their family. However, some children are at risk of serious harm with background factors that cannot be resolved. In the most serious cases a court may need to consider whether the child should be removed from the family by court order and looked after by the local authority, usually in foster care. Children in long-term care have better outcomes if permanent adoption into a new family can be arranged.

KEY POINTS

Characteristics of non-accidental injury:
- Injuries in very young children.
- Explanations that do not match the appearance of the injury, and which change.
- Multiple types and age of injury.
- Injuries that are 'classic' in site or character.
- Delay in presentation.
- Disclosure by the child.

Adolescence is the time between childhood and full maturity and is when growing-up occurs. It is a time of great physical, psychological and social change, and can be a time of considerable stress for adolescents and their parents

Physical changes
- Growth spurt occurs—may feel 'gangly'
- Secondary sex characteristics develop:
  - pubic hair
  - facial hair and testicular enlargement in boys
  - breast enlargement in girls
- Voice deepens in boys
- Girls undergo menarche and become fertile
- Acne may develop
- Gynaecomastia may develop in boys

'Tasks' of adolescence
- Establish sense of identity
- Achieve independence
- Achieve sexual maturity
- Take on adult responsibility
- Develop adult thinking

Psychological problems
- Eating disorders
- Depression
- Self-harm
- Overdosing on medicines
- Suicide

Psychological changes
- Develop insight
- Able to use abstract reasoning
- Develop logical thought
- Able to reason morally, often leading to questioning of parents and awareness of social injustice in the world
- Search for independence
- May be emotional turmoil and conflict
- Experimentation and risk-taking behaviour

Health issues
- Contraception and safe sex
- Acne
- Eating disorders
  - anorexia
  - bulimia
  - obesity
- Chronic illness (diabetes, cystic fibrosis, Crohn's disease, asthma)
- Health promotion
- Issues of consent

Health destructive behaviour
- Alcohol
- Smoking
- Drug use
- Substance abuse
- Accidents
- Unsafe sex
  - sexually transmitted disease
  - unwanted pregnancy
  - teenage pregnancy
- Excessive dieting

Vulnerable adolescents
Certain groups of adolescents are at particular risk of a poor outcome through adolescence and may also have difficulty accessing healthcare They include:
- Those with chronic illness (e.g. diabetes), physical disability or learning difficulties
- The homeless and unemployed
- Victims of physical, emotional or sexual abuse
- Those who are pregnant
- Some ethnic minority groups
- Those from disrupted homes

Social change
- Still dependent on parents financially and for housing
- Greater freedom and flexibility
- Self-motivation and self-discipline expected by school
- Sexual interest and activity increases; most experience some form of sexual activity
- Face leaving school and moving to higher education, work, financial independence or unemployment

Approach to the adolescent
- Adolescence is generally a time of life when illness is rare
- Partly because of this, healthcare facilities for adolescents are poor, often falling between paediatric and adult care
- The low rate of contact with doctors means health promotion must be delivered to the adolescent
- Adolescents may be concerned about confidentiality when seeing their family doctor
- Drop-in clinics can offer immediate advice on health issues, counselling for emotional and personal problems and contraceptive advice
- The way in which health professionals treat adolescents is important

How to treat adolescents
- Take time to listen
- Show respect for their emerging maturity
- Allow them to express their concerns
- Avoid making judgemental statements
- Assure confidentiality (but make it clear there are times when confidentiality must be broken, e.g. after disclosure of ongoing abuse or if others are at risk)
- Respect the need for privacy—offer to see them without their parents

Adolescent harmful health behaviours
Adolescence is naturally a time of increasing independence for young people away from parental supervision. It is normal for young people to experiment with more adult activities and to show some rebellious behaviours. With the right level of support and supervision young people learn about independence in a safe way. There are often difficulties for families in communicating about some of these issues and this period of emotional and physical development is often hard for young people and parents.

Smoking, drug and alcohol abuse

Teenage smoking is increasing, especially among girls. Smoking often becomes a dependency which has lifelong health consequences.

An increasing proportion of teenagers experiment with drug use. Solvent abuse is also common. Young people need age-appropriate support to manage substance abuse.

Harmful drinking behaviours often begin in adolescence. There is a risk of injury through accident, assault and coma. This can be viewed as experimentation behaviour but sometimes represents a self-harming behaviour with more serious background social problems.

Accidents

Road traffic accidents are the leading cause of death in this age group. Alcohol and failure to wear seat belts or crash helmets increase the risks.

Self-harming

Drug overdose is a common cause of admission to hospital in adolescence. This is often a response to a stressful situation linked to family or peer relationship problems and reflects vulnerability and difficulty getting effective support. There is not usually a serious suicidal intent but the overdose may inadvertently result in serious poisoning. Self-harming can also manifest as deliberate soft-tissue cutting or burning behaviours. Young people who self-harm should be seen acutely by mental health professionals to assess level of risk and to arrange ongoing support.

Sexual health issues
Menstrual complaints

Amenorrhoea is often physiological as periods may be very irregular or scanty for months after the onset of menarche. Stress associated with moving schools or exams can disrupt periods, and those undergoing intense athletic training may develop amenorrhoea. Eating disorders and chronic illness can cause amenorrhoea. Pregnancy should also be considered as a cause.

Menorrhagia (heavy periods) and *dysmenorrhoea* (painful menstrual cramps) are common in the first few years after menarche. Treatment includes prostaglandin synthetase inhibitors (e.g. mefenamic acid) to reduce bleeding or the combined oral contraceptive pill to regulate the cycle.

Polycystic ovary syndrome can present in adolescence with the combination of amenorrhoea, obesity, hirsutism and acne. There are later fertility problems.

Unsafe sex

Many adolescents have higher risk-taking sexual behaviours. Provision of easily accessible school-based sexual health services can help by giving confidential health information and improves uptake of contraception and testing for sexually transmitted diseases (STDs). Young people are at higher risk of sexual assault from peers and older adults with greater risk following drug or alcohol use.

Teenage pregnancy

Some 40% of sexually active teenage girls become pregnant within 2 years. The UK has the highest teenage pregnancy rate in Europe. There are increased perinatal risks for the mother and for the baby. Early support to young mothers and their children is important in improving their long-term outcomes.

Abortion

One third of teenage pregnancies are managed by termination of pregnancy. There may be reluctance to seek help, sense of guilt and fears about confidentiality so there is a clear need for sensitive support.

Contraception

Less than 50% use contraception at the time of first having sex. Information and ready access to contraception are important to reduce the rate of teenage pregnancy. Condoms prevent the spread of STDs. The oral contraceptive pill is a reliable method if taken correctly. An alternative is depot (parenteral) hormonal contraception. Intrauterine devices are not usually offered to nulliparous women and carry a risk of pelvic infection. The 'morning-after pill' hormonal contraception can be taken up to 72 hours after unprotected sex but often causes sickness and is less reliable with increasing delay in use.

Sexually transmitted diseases

STDs such as chlamydia, gonorrhoea and herpes are prevalent in the community and increasingly seen in adolescents. Screening for chlamydia by urine polymerase chain reaction (PCR) test is offered at school sexual health clinics.

Eating disorders

Eating disorders are characterized by a fear of being overweight and a distorted body image, so that even extremely wasted individuals feel they are overweight. There may be preoccupation with food and bizarre eating behaviours.

Eating disorders are commoner in girls than boys, and often start as dieting behaviour. The age of onset is becoming younger. Background factors include peer group focus on thin body shape and family history of eating disorders.

Anorexia nervosa

This involves extreme dieting to control weight. There may also be excessive physical activity. In anorexia the body mass index (BMI) reduces below 17.5, with dangerous physical changes below BMI 15. Features include emaciation, amenorrhoea, hair loss and lanugo hair. Bradycardia, hypothermia, hypotension and biochemical derangement develop with extreme malnutrition. The mortality rate for anorexia can be up to 10%. In severe situations admission to hospital may be needed for managed refeeding up to the desired weight; nasogastric feeding may be required. Behavioural modification techniques are used to help to reach a healthy weight. The overall prognosis is good with a multidisciplinary team approach.

Bulimia

This is characterized by bouts of binge eating, followed by purging with laxatives or by inducing vomiting. Oesophagitis, parotid swelling and enamel erosion of the teeth are all signs of chronic vomiting.

KEY POINTS
- Adolescence is a time of rapid physical, psychological and social change.
- Adolescents learn independence but are at risk of harmful risk-taking behaviour.
- Eating disorders are common and need expert management.
- Health workers need to find novel ways of engaging with adolescents, especially vulnerable groups.

Sudden infant death and acute life-threatening events

Aetiology
- Most common cause of death in infants >1 week
- Increased risk if prone, overheated or smoky environment
- Normally previously well babies, sometimes with minor cough or cold
- In 20% an unexpected cause is found at autopsy

Examination
- Found collapsed
- Pale and mottled
- Bradycardia
- Hypotension

Investigations
- Blood sugar
- Infection screen
- CXR and barium swallow
- ECG monitoring
- Metabolic screen

Management of acute life-threatening events
- Cardiopulmonary resuscitation (CPR)
- Admit for observation and investigation
- Train parents to administer CPR
- Home apnoea monitor may relieve anxiety but is of no proven benefit

Differential diagnosis
- Infection
- Gastro-oesophageal reflux
- Neurological abnormality
- Hypoglycaemia (rare)
- Cardiac arrhythmia (rare)
- Inborn error of metabolism (rare)
- Suffocation (rare)
- Non-accidental injury

Acute life-threatening events and SIDS

Sudden infant death syndrome (SIDS) is the sudden death of an infant with no apparent pathological cause on post-mortem. It is commonly known as 'cot death' since typically the death occurs overnight in the baby's cot. It is vital for the family to have a thorough investigation of the sudden death. A detailed case investigation needs a combined approach by a senior paediatrician, social services and police professionals. There is review of the history and clinical examination findings, examination of the scene of death to consider any environmental risk factors and a later meeting to review post-mortem results. It is very important to involve the family in this process to give as full an explanation as possible of the events and what can be understood about their child's death.

Sometimes infants are found in a collapsed state, not breathing and looking grey or mottled, but can be successfully resuscitated. This is referred to as an acute life-threatening event (ALTE) or as 'near-miss cot death'. All of these cases need careful medical and sometimes forensic investigation to try to establish a cause.

SIDS is the commonest cause of death (40%) in infants after the first week of life. The rate varies in different countries, but in the UK is currently 0.45 per 1000. The exact aetiology remains unknown and is probably multifactorial. A triple-risk model has been proposed (see box) which may explain the fact that SIDS peaks between 2 and 4 months, and 90% occur before 6 months of age.

Triple-risk model

- A vulnerable infant with inherent problems of cardiorespiratory control (e.g. the premature infant)
- A critical period of development. (changes in arousal, sleep–wake patterns and metabolism)
- External environmental stressors (e.g. prone sleeping, cigarette smoke, temperature, infection)

In the UK the incidence of SIDS has fallen by over 50% as a result of the 'Back to Sleep' campaign (see box) which advises that babies should be put to sleep on their backs, at the foot of the cot, not overwrapped or overheated. This followed research which established that there is an eightfold increase in SIDS if the child sleeps in the prone position and a twofold risk in the side-lying position. Other risk factors include cigarette smoke in the home, parental alcohol intake and co-sleeping. There is some recent evidence that keeping the baby in the parents' bedroom (but not bed-sharing) and the use of a dummy (pacifier) may be associated with a reduced risk of SIDS. A small number of what initially appear to be SIDS cases may be due to non-accidental injury with atypical history or abnormal findings on post-mortem. In the UK the 'Care of the Next Infant' (CONI) project can provide support to families who have suffered a sudden death in infancy to try to reduce the small possibility of recurrence through advice about risk factors, regular monitoring check-ups and resuscitation training. The use of breathing alarm (apnoea) monitors is controversial but some parents find them reassuring.

Sudden unexpected death in childhood (SUDIC) is a broader category where a child has died unexpectedly from any cause. It is best practice to review all such deaths (e.g. road traffic accidents, acute catastrophic infection) through a multidisciplinary approach so health protection agencies can learn lessons and also to provide as full an explanation as possible to the family.

Acute life threatening events

A large number of infants are admitted to hospital following an apparent acute life-threatening event (ALTE). This may be from an obvious cause such as choking on a bottle feed to unexplained apnoeic episodes or even a 'near-miss cot death' where the child has been successfully resuscitated. All these infants need careful evaluation and usually a period of observation and monitoring in hospital. In difficult cases prolonged cardiac, respiratory, oxygenation and even video analysis may be necessary to establish the sequence of events. Common causes include gastro-oesophageal reflux, infection (e.g. RSV bronchiolitis) and anaemia. Inborn errors of metabolism, seizures and cardiac arrhythmias are more unusual findings.

Parental support must be offered. There is controversy over the role of apnoea monitors, but they may provide parental reassurance in selected cases.

The 'Back to Sleep' campaign

• Place the baby on its back to sleep.
• Do not smoke in the house. Try not to smoke during pregnancy.
• Put the baby in the 'feet to foot' position in the cot, with feet touching the foot of the cot and the head uncovered. This aims to prevent the baby slipping under the covers.
• Do not sleep a baby on a pillow or cushion. Do not use padded cot sides.
• Use any kind of firm mattress.
• Do not let the baby get too hot or cold. Use a sheet and layers of blankets appropriate for the temperature rather than a duvet. Keep room temperature 16–20°C
• Do not sleep in the same bed as the baby if you smoke, have taken alcohol or drugs, or are very tired. Never sleep on a sofa with your baby.
• Seek medical advice if your baby seems ill.
  For further details see http://www.fsid.org.uk

KEY POINTS

• SIDS is the commonest cause of death in infancy outside the neonatal period.
• Following the advice of the 'Back to Sleep' Campaign can dramatically reduce the risk.
• Acute life threatening events (ALTEs) need careful evaluation as they may be a precursor of sudden death in infancy.
• SIDS has a multifactorial aetiology, which is the subject of ongoing research.

There are many situations in paediatric medicine which involve ethical questions. Ethics are the moral values that people hold which enable them to understand whether a judgement is right or wrong. These values usually start to develop from the early experiences of childhood and continue to develop right through into adult years. The values involve a sense of consideration for others, the law, personal conscience, religious beliefs, cultural beliefs and personal experience.

Cornerstones of medical ethics

- Autonomy (self-determination)
- Beneficence (doing good)
- Non-malificence (not doing harm)
- Justice (fairness and equality)

Important concepts that guide ethical decisions in critical care

- **Human rights—the right to life:** There are different views on whether life must always be sustained in all circumstances but there is a general view that life must be respected and not harmed. There are some situations where the vast majority of people would agree that prolonging life at all costs is wrong (such as following diagnosis of brain death) and the law will support a decision to stop treatment and allow death to occur.
- **Acts of commission and omission:** The difference between a decision that actively ends life and a decision to withhold or discontinue intervention that is prolonging life
- **Quality of life:** Most people believe this is important and is significantly impaired if:
  - life is dependent on invasive medical support
  - there is chronic distress
  - there is severe impairment of consciousness.

Consent, autonomy and confidentiality

In general treatment should always be given with a patient's consent. However, this is not always possible with young children. Children are unlike adults in that other people (usually parents) are legally allowed to make decisions on their behalf.

Very young children are not able to understand or communicate a decision so their parents or carers act as advocates in agreeing to treatment. Usually there is no conflict of interest but this is not always the case. A parent may hold a view that is different from that of the healthcare team—they may wish to prevent a specific life-saving treatment being given, despite medical advice. There are also some situations where parents may disagree with a request to withdraw life-sustaining treatment. Usually such disagreement can be resolved through sensitive communication or by offering an independent second opinion, but occasionally it is necessary for doctors to ask a court to give a judgement on whether treatment should be given.

As children get older and gain understanding they should be more involved in decisions about their care. It is best practice to seek consent from children as well as their parents. It is generally believed that young people are best supported by involving their parents in issues relating to their health. They are usually encouraged to do this. However, there may be situations where the young person is reluctant to involve a parent and this may be harmful if they then fail to seek medical care. An example of this is an adolescent girl who wants to request contraception but is fearful that the doctor will inform her parent. If the doctor considers that the young person is mature enough to understand the implications of a treatment then the parent does not have to be informed. This level of competence is sometimes referred to as 'Gillick competence' after a legal test case ruling.

Ethics in critical care—withdrawal of intensive care

It is not always clear whether it is right to start, or to continue, life-supporting intensive care. If a neonate is born at the very limit of prematurity (22–23 weeks gestation) then some people would consider it wrong to proceed with intensive care given the extremely poor chance of survival. If a child has severe chronic ill health with no cure available then it may be wrong to pursue repeated episodes of intensive care. If a child has severe brain injury then it may be right to withdraw ventilator support to allow them to die. It is important to consider whether a situation might arise in the future when such a decision may need to be made for a child. There are situations where this can be discussed beforehand with the family and, in some instances, the child may be involved in the decision.

These decisions are very difficult and require doctors to work together with families to ensure that families have full understanding of the issues of prognosis, pain and suffering, and potential quality of life if treatment is continued. It is important that all members of the medical and nursing team are able to raise any concerns and any disagreement is resolved.

End-of-life care

Actively supporting children and families through palliative care is very important. Care of the dying patient through a specialist paediatric multidisciplinary palliative care team can achieve immense benefits in terms of symptom control, care at home, family support and maintaining a child-centred approach. Palliative care teams help many children with life-limiting neurological, oncological, metabolic, congenital and other disorders, sometimes over a period of many years.

KEY POINTS

- Ethical decisions usually do not need to be made rapidly—there is time for full consultation.
- It is usually wrong to make decisions that conflict with the views of parents.
- All relevant staff members must be involved in discussions before a decision is made.
- Discuss all options with parents so that they know that all the possible courses of treatment have been considered.
- A child who is mature enough should be involved in ethical decisions.
- Adolescents may receive treatment without parental knowledge, provided they are deemed mature enough to appreciate its consequences
- Where dispute persists between clinical staff and parents, the courts should be asked to make a final decision.

Core self-assessment case studies: questions

Case 1: A vomiting baby

A 5-week-old baby has been vomiting for the last 48 hours. Initially he was keeping some feeds down but now he is vomiting after every feed. He was breast-fed initially but for the last week has been given formula milk via a bottle because his mother, who is only 17, developed a breast abscess and decided to stop breast-feeding.

1 You are worried about this baby, who seems quite ill. What further information do you need from the history?

You examine the baby. His temperature is 36.8 °C. He has sunken eyes, a slightly sunken fontanelle and dry mucous membranes. The nappy is dry and empty. His pulse is 160 beats/min, blood pressure is 70/40 and his capillary refill time 3 seconds. He weighs 3.0 kg. He is irritable. As you examine him he vomits milk on to your shoe.

2 Do you think he is dehydrated? If so, to what degree?

3 His mother is carrying her child health record (red book). How can you establish exactly the degree of dehydration?

Following your examination you decide to admit the child and undertake some blood tests. These are the results:

- Sodium 130 mmol/L ↓
- Potassium 2.8 mmol/L ↓
- Chloride 90 mmol/L ↓
- Bicarbonate 32 mmol/L ↑
- Creatinine 90 mmol/L ↑
- Urea 6.7 mmol/L ↑
- Glucose 5.5 mmol/L ⁼
- pH 7.53 ↑
- Pco_2 5.5 KPa ⁼
- Po_2 14 KPa ⁼
- Base excess +7 mmol/L

4 Which of the following is the most likely diagnosis?

- Acute renal failure
- Inborn error of metabolism
- Aspirin poisoning
- Administration of hyperconcentrated milk feeds
- Pyloric stenosis
- Severe gastroenteritis
- Diabetic ketoacidosis

Your senior colleague reviews the child and decides that he is 8% dehydrated and needs rehydration.

5 What fluid would you use to rehydrate him and by what route? Can you calculate his fluid deficit in millilitres?

6 What is the definitive treatment for this child?

Case 2: Developmental delay

Suzie is 24 months old. Her health visitor has referred her for a check-up as she is concerned that Suzie is not yet beginning to talk. Suzie's mother is not too worried, as her mother told her that she was a slow developer herself.

You take a developmental history and discover that Suzie walked at 13 months, and is now able to run. You settle down to play with Suzie and find that she can build a tower of three bricks when she is shown how. She readily takes a crayon but does not know how to scribble. She babbles happily to herself but does not have any words yet. Her mother tells you that she waves bye-bye, eats with her fingers and drinks from a bottle. She has been offered a spoon, but has shown no interest in using it.

1 What are the four developmental areas that you should assess?

2 What do you think of the milestones she has attained?

3 What are possible causes of Suzie's developmental delay?

4 What is important to look for in your history and physical examination?

5 Should you consider doing any investigations?

6 What is your next step?

Case 3: A wheezy child

An 18-month-old child presents with his first episode of wheeze. He is pyrexial and has shortness of breath with some subcostal recession. Wheeze is heard all over his chest.

1 Which of the following diagnoses are most likely?

- Asthma
- Inhaled foreign body
- Bronchiolitis
- Croup
- Whooping cough

2 If you were considering asthma as a likely diagnosis, what family history may be relevant?

3 If you were considering bronchiolitis as a likely diagnosis, what diagnostic test would you perform?

The child is admitted to the ward. Over the next few hours the shortness of breath settles with treatment. The wheeze remains intermittently present; worse prior to each treatment.

4 What treatment is likely to have been given?

The next day the child is better and is discharged home. He is reviewed in the outpatient department 6 weeks later, during which time he has had two further episodes of shortness of breath. He coughs most nights. You decide to prescribe treatment.

5 What would you prescribe and what would you tell his parents about administering it?

On further review 3 months later he is well, but still coughing at night several nights a week. He has been unable to attend nursery on a few occasions.

6 What further treatment would you consider?

Case 4: Headaches

A 12-year-old boy comes to you complaining of recurrent headaches. He has had five episodes over the last 4 months. They started around the time he began high school, which coincided with his parents' divorce. Each time they began with a throbbing pain that was usually focused on the right side of his head. On one occasion he vomited. On each occasion he came home from school, took some paracetamol and lay down. He is not happy at school and is finding it hard academically and socially.

You examine him carefully. His blood pressure is 110/67 and pulse is 64. He has no neurological signs.

1 What diagnoses do you consider?

2 What features make you consider that migraine is a probable diagnosis? What else would you look for in the history?

3 What features in a history of headache would make you worry that he might have raised intracranial pressure?
4 What treatment would you consider?
5 When would you consider requesting investigations?

Case 5: Joint swelling

You are asked to see a 5-year-old girl who has been unwell for several weeks and has had an intermittent fever. She has complained of swelling in her knees and some stiffness in her joints in the mornings. On examination she looks pale and tired with a red swollen left knee.

1 What else would you like to establish from the history?

She is reviewed by your senior colleague who comes up with a differential diagnosis of the following:

- Osteomyelitis
- Chronic fatigue syndrome
- Leukaemia
- Juvenile chronic arthritis
- Trauma

2 Which do you think is the most likely diagnosis?

Blood tests are performed which show the following:

- Haemoglobin 9.6 g/dL ↓
- White cell count 12×10^9/L =
- Platelets 500×10^9/L ↑
- Reticulocytes 1% =
- Mean corpuscular volume (MCV) 80 fL =
- Mean corpuscular haemoglobin (MCH) 23 pg ↓
- C-reactive protein (CRP) 32 ↑
- Erythrocyte sedimentation rate (ESR) 45 mm/h ↑

3 What do these blood tests show?
4 What treatment would you advise?

Case 6: Failure to thrive

The health visitor has asked you to see an 8-month-old baby girl as she has not been gaining weight recently. Her weight at the age of 6 months was on the 25th centile and it is now on the 2nd. She had an episode of gastroenteritis when she was 26 weeks old. She has recovered but still has loose stools. Her mother says that she has become rather irritable, and is not feeding as well as she used to.

On examination her length is on the 50th centile, as is her head circumference. She looks thin, and her abdomen protrudes somewhat. Otherwise her physical examination is normal.

1 What are the possible causes of her poor weight gain?
2 What might suggest an organic rather than a psychosocial cause?
3 How would you manage this baby?
4 What investigations might you consider?
5 If your investigations come back normal, what would your next step be?

Case 7: Heart murmur

You are asked to see a baby girl in the Emergency Department. She was born 8 weeks ago after an uncomplicated pregnancy. She has had increasing difficulty completing bottle feeds, sometimes taking up to 45 minutes per feed. On examination she looks breathless. She has a heart murmur.

1 What else would you look for on examination to establish whether the murmur is the cause of her symptoms?

The murmur is loudest at the left sternal edge and radiates to the apex. It has a harsh rasping quality and is throughout systole. The heart sounds are normal. A chest radiograph shows cardiomegaly and plethoric lung fields.

2 What is the likely cardiac diagnosis?

You arrange for a cardiac echocardiogram on this child. It confirms the diagnosis. The child is commenced on diuretic medication. A corrective operation is planned for when the child is older.

3 What advice would you give the child's parents regarding dental treatment?

Case 8: Obesity

Kirsty, who is 10 years old, comes to see you with her mother as she has been putting on a good deal of weight. They think the problem started 2 years ago, and she now weighs 80 kg and is 148 cm tall. She is in her last year at primary school and is by far the tallest girl in the class. She has been an excellent pupil to date and has happily gone to school in the past, but over the last term she has begun to refuse to go. She says that she does not like it anymore as children have started to tease her because of her weight.

Her mother, who is overweight herself, has been trying to encourage her to eat fruit and vegetables, and has also tried to encourage her to be more active, but Kirsty resists as she is ridiculed when she does so. Mrs Hare recognizes that Kirsty's lifestyle is not ideal, but does not feel that it fully explains her weight problem. She is becoming convinced that Kirsty has a glandular problem.

1 You are sure that Kirsty does not have a hormonal or glandular cause for her obesity. How can you be so sure?
2 What is important to ask about in the history?
3 What do you look for on physical examination?
4 Is it worthwhile doing any investigations?
5 Her mother asks you if you can reassure her that Kirsty simply has puppy fat. What do you say?
6 What help can you offer Kirsty?

Case 9: Abdominal pain

A 4-year-old girl called Emily is taken by her parents to the family doctor. She has been non-specifically unwell since she had a viral illness a few weeks before. Her mother is worried because she has been complaining of tummy ache. She has been wetting the bed again, having been dry at night since the age of 20 months.

1 What investigation would you do in the first instance to investigate her abdominal pain and bedwetting?

Emily's mother collects a clean-catch urine sample and takes it to the doctor's surgery. The doctor performs a dipstick test and then sends the urine to the lab. The results are as follows:

- Dipstick:
  - Specific gravity 1010
  - Leucocytes +++
  - Protein ++
  - Nitrites –ve
  - Glucose ++++
- Laboratory results:
  - White cells 10–20
  - Red cells: none
  - Gram stain –ve
  - Culture: mixed growth

2 How do you interpret the dipstick result?
3 How do you interpret the laboratory result?

When the doctor rings the family to discuss the result, he finds that Emily has become more unwell, with severe abdominal pain and has been vomiting all night. He decides to visit at home.

When he arrives at the home Emily is dehydrated and semi-conscious. He calls an ambulance. As a precaution he checks her blood glucose and finds that it is 28 mmol/L. He telephones ahead to the hospital to warn them.

4 What is the diagnosis? What treatment will she require when she reaches hospital?

Extended self-assessment case studies: questions

Case 1: A short girl

Tracey is 10 years old and is the shortest girl in her class. Her height is 122 cm and is on the 0.4th centile.

1 *What would you look for in your history and physical examination?*
2 *Would you carry out any investigations and if so which?*

A radiograph of her wrist shows she has a bone age of 9 years.

3 *What does this mean?*

You request a karyotype. The result shows that her chromosome complement is 45XO.

4 *What is her diagnosis?*
5 *What treatment is available for her?*

Case 2: Constipation

Billie is 6 years old. He has been experiencing abdominal pain and has been passing hard stools with difficulty. Last night he had some rectal bleeding.

1 *What is his diagnosis?*
2 *How would you treat him and how long for?*
3 *What would make you think of Hirschsprung's disease as a diagnosis?*

Some months later he returns. His mother is distressed because he has been soiling his underpants.

4 *What is the likely explanation?*
5 *What is the difference between soiling and encopresis?*
6 *What is his prognosis?*

Case 3: Cough and fever

Jenny is 3 years old. She has had a cold for a few days. Since yesterday she has had a fever of 39.5° and has been coughing through the night. You examine her and find that her throat is inflamed, her tympanic membranes are pink and she has some wheezing and coarse crepitations throughout her chest.

1 *What additional signs would you look for to check whether she might have a lower respiratory tract infection?*
2 *How reliable is auscultation and percussion in a child of this age?*
3 *What investigations would you consider?*

A chest radiograph shows signs of localized consolidation in the right middle lobe pneumonia.

4 *What is the likely causative organism?*

Case 4: Fits, faints and funny spells

Tommy is 18 months old. For some months now he has been throwing temper tantrums. In the last week these have changed in character and on two occasions he has stopped breathing, turned blue and then gone limp. By the time emergency services have been called he has recovered. Tommy has had no medical problems in the past and is developing normally.

1 *What is the differential diagnosis?*
2 *How can you distinguish breath-holding spells from other fits, faints and funny spells?*
3 *If you were not sure that these were breath-holding spells, what might you ask the family to do?*

4 *How would you advise the family to manage breath-holding spells?*
5 *What is the prognosis for breath-holding spells?*

Case 5: A jaundiced baby

You are asked to review a full-term baby on the postnatal ward who is 12 hours old. The midwife is concerned that the baby looks jaundiced. You go to see the baby who is jaundiced and has yellow sclera but is alert and has just completed a breast feed. You review the history including the history of the recent pregnancy.

1 *What information do you need to know about the mother and the pregnancy?*
2 *What immediate tests should you perform on the baby?*

The serum bilirubin comes back from the lab as 200 μmol/L.

3 *What will you do with the bilirubin result?*
4 *What treatment is mandatory?*
5 *What other treatment might you consider? What would influence your decision?*
6 *The serum bilirubin peaked at 450 μmol/L on day 4 of life but the child recovers well after appropriate therapy. You arrange to see them in the outpatient clinic at 2–3 weeks of age. What tests might this child need as an outpatient?*

Case 6: A baby with suspected cyanosis

You are asked to see a baby who is 24 hours old. He is the third baby of the family. Mother is of African origin and has insulin-dependent diabetes. The baby was breast-feeding well until a few hours ago and has no signs of respiratory distress. The mother is worried about the baby's colour and think he looks 'blue around the lips'.

1 *What will you look for on examination?*
2 *What simple bedside investigation can help make a diagnosis of cyanotic CHD?*
3 *What would be your immediate management if the examination and investigations suggest CHD?*
4 *A routine blood test shows the haemoglobin to be 22 g/dL. Is this relevant?*
5 *What do you think the cardiac diagnosis might be?*

Case 7: A swelling in the groin

A 9-year-old boy is at home with his parents when he suddenly complains of a pain in his right groin. He has been playing football all afternoon. As a baby he had a hydrocele on the right side of his scrotum but this disappeared when he was about 12 months old. His father has a look at his groin area and noticed the right side of his scrotum is swollen and extremely tender. He telephones the family doctor for advice as to what he should do next.

1 *List four conditions that should be in the GP's differential diagnosis for this presentation?*
2 *What features on examination will differentiate between them?*
3 *If the boy had complained of a headache, a swollen face and a fever in the preceding days, what other condition might you consider?*

The GP sends the boy to the local hospital for review by a paediatric surgeon. The surgeon finds a tense red swelling in the right scrotum and inguinal canal. It is difficult to 'get above it' and the testis is not easily palpable on that side. The swelling is not reducible.

4 *What is the diagnosis and what is the treatment?*
5 *What is the danger of delaying treatment?*

Case 8: A collapsed child

You are walking home one day when you pass a group of schoolchildren at a bus stop. One of them is coughing and seems to be getting into a panic. As you approach he falls to the ground clutching at his neck. His friends scream and you rush over to help. As you approach the boy he is becoming pale and cyanosed. You can hear an inspiratory 'whistling' noise and he is finding it increasingly hard to breathe.

1 *What immediate actions should you undertake?*

After a further 1 minute he becomes unconscious and slumps over. You notice he has a half-open bag of peanuts in his hand and there are peanuts all around the ground on the pavement.

2 *Now what should you do?*

After a further 2 minutes your intervention is successful and he starts to breathe again.

3 *Now what should you do?*
4 *What investigations might be performed once he reaches hospital?*

Case 9: A child with vomiting and altered conscious level

A 7-year-old boy is brought to the Emergency Department with a 1-day history of worsening vomiting. Over the last few hours parents report that he has been much less responsive and is now not talking but only making moaning noises. He has had bedwetting over the last 2 weeks having previously been dry at night from age 3. On examination he is pale, dehydrated, making laboured respiratory effort, rate of breathing is 50/min. He is lying in his mother's arms, opens his eyes when his name is called, movement is reduced but he will move his arm away from a painful stimulus.

1 *Is there a need for any resuscitation intervention?*
2 *What is the Glasgow Coma Score of this patient?*
3 *What level of monitoring is required?*
4 *Which of the following diagnoses is most likely?*
   a Ingestion of poisonous drug/ chemical
   b Intracerebral haemorrhage
   c Meningitis
   d Diabetic ketoacidosis
   e Gastroenteritis
5 *What investigations should be performed urgently?*
6 *Describe the management over the next few hours*

Case 10: A 3-month-old baby with bruises

A 3 month old baby boy is referred by the GP who noticed a number of bruises when the baby was seen for their routine immunizations. The baby attends with both parents. There is a 1-cm circular bruise to the left cheek and two similar-size bruises to the abdomen. The baby is a little quiet and it is mentioned that his feeds have reduced that day but he is otherwise well. There is no history of any injury.

1 *What further history is needed?*
2 *What specific signs should be checked on examination?*
3 *What investigations should be performed?*
4 *What safeguarding process should occur?*

Case 11: A 14-year-old girl with cystic fibrosis

A 14-year-old girl is seen for routine review in the cystic fibrosis clinic. She was diagnosed in the neonatal period and has been under regular follow-up since infancy. She has been well over the last 2 months with her only current respiratory symptom a persistent mild cough. She has good exercise tolerance and participates in sports at school. She is taking a large number of oral and nebulized medications but manages to adhere to the regimen and her physiotherapy.

1 *What key features in clinic give a guide to her current health and prognosis?*
2 *What issues are likely to arise over the next 5 years as she reaches adult age?*

Case 12: A 12-year-old girl with progressive tiredness

A 12-year-old girl is referred by her general practitioner with a history of excessive tiredness. She was previously fit and well and performed well in a competitive athletics club. Over the last 3 months she has had difficulty in participating in normal school and home activities. She complains of feeling tired shortly after starting any exercise and has stopped doing all sports. On return from school she has been going to bed very early in the evening. Her overnight sleep pattern has been disrupted. Her appetite is reduced. She has some pain symptoms affecting muscles of legs and lower back. Over the last 6 weeks she has not attended a full school day and has missed a total of 4 weeks completely as she has felt too tired to attend on waking. She has struggled to maintain contact with her friends and has missed several social events.

1 *What illness problems need to be considered in this situation?*
2 *What further history is important?*
3 *What investigations should be performed?*
4 *What management approach should be used?*

Core self-assessment case studies: answers

Case 1: A vomiting baby

1 You need to establish the cause of the vomiting. Is it associated with diarrhoea, which would make gastroenteritis more likely, or is it associated with constipation, which may suggest a bowel obstruction? Is the vomiting bile stained, which suggests a serious bowel obstruction, or is it just curdled milk? Is the vomiting minor posseting, suggestive of gastro-oesophageal reflux, or is it projectile, as occurs in pyloric stenosis? Finally, the baby has recently changed feeds so you might want to ask how this young mother is making up the feeds—non-sterile water may cause gastroenteritis, or over-concentrated feeds may cause electrolyte imbalance.

2 This child shows features of moderate dehydration (5–10%), with a sunken fontanelle, dry lips, tachycardia and slightly long capillary refill time, but without signs of shock. The dry nappy suggests he may not be passing urine, but this needs to be established from the history.

3 Look for a recent weight. In fact this baby weighed 3.3 kg a week ago. He has therefore lost 300 g. If we assume all this weight loss is due to fluid loss, this represents 9% dehydration.

4 Pyloric stenosis. There is a metabolic alkalosis and hypokalaemia due to depletion of H^+ in the vomit. The timing (4–6 weeks), male sex, increasing vomiting and constipation, lack of bile and irritability are typical features. Acute renal failure would show a higher creatinine and hyperkalaemia. Concentrated feeds would cause hypernatraemia. Most of these conditions cause acidosis. The normal glucose excludes diabetic ketoacidosis. This child is too young to have accidentally ingested aspirin. Aspirin poisoning typically causes a respiratory alkalosis due to hyperventilation, then progresses to a metabolic acidosis.

5 Normally, oral rehydration solution is the safest way to rehydrate this degree of dehydration, but as the child is likely to have pyloric stenosis this will not be absorbed. Intravenous dextrose–saline fluids are indicated, with added potassium to correct the hyperkalaemia.

If this child is 8% dehydrated and weighs 3 kg then his fluid deficit is approximately 8% of 3 L. For this child, this would be $(3300\,mL /100) \times 8 = 264\,mL$.

The fluid prescription should include the child's maintenance fluid requirement and this deficit, given over 24 hours. The maintenance fluid requirement is 100 mL/kg (for the first 10 kg), which $3.3 \times 100 = 330\,mL$.

The total fluids (over 24 hours) is therefore $330 + 264 = 594\,mL$ (= approx. 25 mL/h).

6 This child has pyloric stenosis. Examination of a palpable mass in the epigastric area and visible peristalsis over the stomach after a test feed will confirm the diagnosis. An ultrasound scan may show a thickened, elongated pyloric muscle. The child must be carefully rehydrated prior to the definitive operation, which is Ramstedt's pyloromyotomy.
See Chapters 5, 29 and 30 for further details.

Case 2: Developmental delay

1 The four developmental areas are:
- Gross motor: walking, running
- Fine motor: building a tower, scribbling
- Speech and language: babble and words
- Social skills: waving bye-bye, eating and drinking

2 Suzie has significant developmental delay in all areas other than her gross motor skills, which are appropriate for her age. Her fine motor skills are delayed—at the age of 2 years she should be able to build a tower, and scribble freely. Her language skills are delayed—first words appear at around 12 months. Her social skills are also delayed—finger feeding starts at around 7 months and waving bye-bye at 9 months. By 15 months she should have managed a spoon and a cup. This degree of delay is very worrying and suggests that she is likely to have a significant learning disability.

3 The possible causes of Suzie's developmental picture include:
- Idiopathic causes
- Central nervous system malformation
- Chromosomal abnormalities
- Neurodegenerative disorders
- Pre-, peri- or postnatal natal injury
- Metabolic defects

4 When you take your history it is important to obtain details about any perinatal events, as this may give clues to a pre- or postnatal cause. A family history of consanguinity or developmental problems in other children would suggest a genetic cause.

Pointers in the physical examination include dysmorphic signs, which would suggest a genetic defect, chromosome anomaly or teratogenic effect. Microcephaly would suggest a central neurological cause, fetal alcohol syndrome or intrauterine infection. It is worth looking for neurocutaneous signs and hepatosplenomegaly, which would point to a metabolic disorder.

5 The most common 'cause' is idiopathic and, if there are no significant findings in the history or physical examination, it is unlikely that you will come to a diagnosis. However, chromosome analysis, thyroid function tests and a urine screen for metabolic defects are usually obtained. Any child with speech and language delay requires a hearing test.

6 Suzie needs a full developmental assessment. This is usually carried out by a multidisciplinary team consisting of a physiotherapist, occupational therapist, speech and language therapist, psychologist, paediatrician and health visitor. Appropriate input will be provided to help promote her development.
See Chapters 3 and 62 for further details.

Case 3: A wheezy child

1 Asthma and bronchiolitis are both possible. A child this age is at risk of inhaling a foreign body as they are inquisitive and put small objects in their mouth. A foreign body will either cause airway obstruction leading to choking, stridor and cyanosis, or if inhaled into one main bronchus may cause unilateral wheeze. Fever is less likely. Croup causes a characteristic cough and stridor but no wheeze. Whooping cough presents with coughing and sometimes vomiting but not wheeze.

Bronchiolitis due to respiratory syncytial virus (RSV) infection is very common in the first 2 years of life. There may be a fever. Asthma does not cause fever, but may be triggered by a viral upper respiratory tract infection.

2 You should establish if there is a family history of atopy—asthma, hay fever or eczema in siblings or parents suggest this. Does anybody smoke in the house? Are there any pets in the home?

3 A nasopharyngeal aspirate or swab for RSV immunofluorescence, which can identify the presence of RSV or other respiratory viruses. A chest radiograph may be helpful if there is diagnostic uncertainty or if the child is very ill.

4 The response to treatment followed by recurrence suggests reactive airways disease (asthma) which is responding to bronchodilators such as short-acting beta-agonists (e.g. salbutamol). These may be administered by inhaler (using a spacer device) or by nebulizer.

5 The child probably needs an inhaled beta-agonist such as salbutamol. It is important that this is given via a spacer device as this child is too young to use a metered dose inhaler directly. As he is coughing most nights the bronchodilator should be given regularly at bedtime.

6 He responds to the short-acting bronchodilators but is having regular symptoms despite these. Low-dose inhaled corticosteroids should be given regularly for a trial period to reduce airway inflammation and gain symptom control.

See Chapters 23, 24 and 26 for further details.

Case 4: Headaches

1 The most likely diagnoses are tension headaches or migraine. Tension headaches are more common than migraine, and it certainly sounds like this boy is stressed, having to contend with a new school and his parents' divorce. However, the pain in tension headaches is classically 'band-like'. Other causes of headache include raised intracranial pressure from any cause, dental caries, infections such as sinusitis and eye strain. If he had frequently used non-steroidal analgesics you might consider analgesic headaches.

2 Migraine is a possible diagnosis, particularly as the headaches are one-sided, and as he has vomited on at least one occasion. Features that would reinforce this diagnosis include a history of aura, nausea, a positive family history and a history of travel sickness.

3 You would be concerned that he might have raised intracranial pressure if any of the following symptoms are present:
- pain is worse on lying down
- actual regression in his academic achievements
- hypertension
- papilloedema
- focal neurological signs

4 The first-line treatment for his headaches is rest and simple analgesia. You should enquire sensitively into his family and social situation. You might suggest that he confides in someone—a mentor or teacher at school—or even refer him for counselling. As you consider migraine as a diagnosis, you could suggest that he avoids cheese, chocolate and nuts. If the attacks become more frequent or severe in the future, prophylaxis with beta-blockers or pizotifen is a possibility.

5 Imaging of the brain by CT scan or MRI is only indicated if there are signs of raised intracranial pressure or focal neurological signs, or if headaches persist and are not responsive to normal analgesia.

See Chapter 39 for further details.

Case 5: Joint swelling

1 It is important to establish the duration of her symptoms and whether the pain and swelling has been continuous or recurrent. Has there been any history of trauma or any grazes that might have introduced infection? Has she lost any weight? Are there any other systemic symptoms that might make a malignancy more likely?

2 Juvenile idipathic arthritis. This often presents in an insidious way with hot painful joints which flare up and then settle spontaneously. Systemic symptoms (weight loss, lethargy and recurrent fever) are common.

3 There is a normocytic anaemia with low reticulocyte count suggestive of chronic illness. The high CRP, high ESR and elevated platelets suggest an inflammatory process. The normal white cell count and absence of blast cells makes leukaemia unlikely.

4 In the first instance non-steroidal anti-inflammatory drugs (e.g. ibuprofen) should be used. If the diagnosis of juvenile idiopathic arthritis (either systemic type or pauciarticular type) is confirmed, then disease-modifying drugs such as an immunosuppressant may be needed. Non-drug therapy with physiotherapy and sometimes splinting is advised.

See Chapters 43 and 44 for further details.

Case 6: Failure to thrive

1 The most common reasons for poor weight gain are 'psychosocial'. However, you need to consider the following in your differential diagnosis:
- lactose intolerance (secondary to her gastroenteritis)
- occult infection, e.g. urinary tract infection
- coeliac disease
- cystic fibrosis

2 This baby has loose stools and a protruding abdomen, which should raise your suspicion that she may have an organic cause. Problems in any organ system can be associated with poor weight gain so she needs a thorough history and physical examination, especially focusing on evidence of chest infections, heart murmur, vomiting, recurrent fever, developmental delay, hepatosplenomegaly and neurological signs.

It is important too to look for non-organic symptoms (rather than consider this as a diagnosis of exclusion). Enquire about eating difficulties, difficulties in the home, limitations in the parents, disturbed attachment between mother and child, and maternal depression or psychiatric disorder. Uncommonly, neglect might be a factor.

3 This baby has had an episode of gastroenteritis. It is not uncommon for lactose intolerance to develop due to the enzyme lactase being 'stripped off' by the inflammation. You could check her stool for low pH and sugar-reducing substances. Alternatively it is acceptable to give her a trial of lactose-free formula. She should begin to gain weight rapidly if she is lactose intolerant.

4 The combination of loose stools, poor weight gain and irritability around the time of introduction of wheat products suggests coeliac disease and she therefore requires coeliac antibodies to be measured with confirmation by jejunal biopsy. Another important cause of malabsorption, even though she has not experienced chest infections, is cystic fibrosis and a sweat test is also required. Other investigations usually considered include a full blood count, creatinine and electrolytes, fecal elastase, liver function tests and urine for analysis and culture.

5 If investigations were normal you would be more concerned that there might be psychosocial factors. You should discuss this with the mother, and also suggest that the health visitor paid another home visit to observe a meal and see the interaction around feeding and how the baby eats. You could admit her to hospital, but this is often less helpful. Depending on what the issues are, you might involve the GP, refer to a dietitian, suggest placement in a nursery or involve social services.

See Chapters 8 and 30 for further details.

Case 7: Heart murmur

1 Examine for signs of heart failure (tachypnoea, tachycardia, hepatomegaly, sweating). Respiratory causes such as pneumonia are excluded by the lack of crackles, cough or wheeze and the absence of fever.

2 The nature of the murmur and the breathlessness suggest a left-to-right shunt through a ventricular septal defect.

3 The left-to-right shunt across the ventricular septal defect means that the child is at risk of bacterial endocarditis. Although antibiotic prophylaxis is no longer recommended it is important that parents are advised to keep their child's teeth and gums healthy, to visit a dentist regularly and to avoid body piercing when she is older.

See Chapters 19 and 20 for further details.

Case 8: Obesity

1 Kirsty is tall for her age and also clearly has no learning disability. She therefore has 'simple' or nutritional obesity. Children with a genetic or syndromic cause for their obesity tend to be short, dysmorphic and have learning difficulties. Hormonal causes are rare, and children show poor growth in height as they put on weight.

2 Even though you may not be looking for a cause for Kirsty's obesity, it is important to take a good history. Asthma is more common in obese children and can contribute to a lack of exercise. Sleep apnoea is quite common and you should ask about snoring, cessation of breathing at night and lethargy during the day. A family history of obesity, adult-onset diabetes and cardiovascular disease is relevant.

3 It is important to look for acanthosis nigricans—a dark velvety change in the skin in the neck, axillae and knuckles—as this indi-

cates that she may well already have insulin resistance. Her blood pressure should also be checked.

4 As it is so unlikely that Kirsty has a medical cause for her obesity it is unnecessary to carry out investigations to make a diagnosis. However, you might consider checking a fasting lipid screen, liver function tests and an oral glucose tolerance test as she is at high risk for co-morbidity.

5 Unfortunately you cannot reassure Kirsty and her mother that this is 'puppy fat'. She is at high risk of adult obesity, which is compounded by the family history. You can, however, tell her that if she can only hold her weight steady that she will slim down as she is only 10 and is likely to have a good deal more growth before she reaches adult height.

6 Kirsty needs help in changing her lifestyle. She needs to engage with someone who can encourage her to eat a balanced, healthy diet and be more active. Crash diets are to be discouraged as they tend to lead to a rebound in weight gain, and are potentially damaging in children.

See Chapter 17 for further details.

Case 9: Abdominal pain

1 A urine sample should be obtained and sent for microscopy and culture.

2 The presence of leucocytes and protein are non-specific. The absence of nitrites makes a urinary tract infection unlikely. There is glycosuria.

3 The microscopy is inconclusive. To diagnose a urinary tract infection there should be >50 white cells and a pure growth of bacteria. The negative Gram stain and mixed growth may reflect contamination.

4 Diabetic ketoacidosis (DKA). She has developed type 1 diabetes and her polydipsia and polyuria led to the secondary enuresis. DKA is sometimes mistaken for non-specific abdominal pain or even an acute surgical abdomen.

She will be significantly dehydrated due to the vomiting and the osmotic diuretic effect of persistent glycosuria. She is likely to be acidotic. The treatment priority for the hospital Emergency Department is to rehydrate her. A nasogastric tube should be passed to empty the stomach to reduce the risk of aspiration secondary to gastric paresis. Once stabilized, she will need to commence insulin to reduce her blood glucose concentration.

See Chapters 18 and 28 for further details.

Extended self-assessment case studies: answers

Case 1: A short girl

1
- Tracey needs a full history and clinical examination as poor growth can accompany any chronic condition. Most chronic illnesses will be evident, but inflammatory bowel disease and chronic renal failure can be occult. Look for signs of hypothyroidism and any dysmorphic features.
- Take a birth history, as babies small for gestational age can have reduced growth potential. A psychosocial history is essential as emotional neglect and abuse can stunt growth and social difficulties can result from short stature.
- Find out if there is a history of maturational delay in the family (mother's age of menarche is particularly relevant). Obtain parental heights so you can calculate the target range for the child's.
- Previous growth measurements are critical, as fall-off in growth would suggest a medical problem.

2 If there has been a fall-off in growth, investigations are always required. They are also indicated if the child is extremely short (height below 0.4th centile). The following need to be considered: full blood count and plasma viscosity, urea and electrolytes, coeliac antibodies, thyroxine and TSH, karyotype, radiograph of the wrist for bone age. Growth hormone stimulation tests should be considered if the growth velocity is reduced on serial measurements or the height is extremely short.

3 The bone age is slightly delayed. In growth hormone deficiency and hypothyroidism a more significant delay is seen. The commonest cause of delayed bone age is simple maturational delay.

4 Tracey has Turner's syndrome. The diagnosis is usually made at a younger age because of short stature. It is also commonly identified before birth at amniocentesis or ultrasound. The classical dysmorphic features are not always present.

5 Tracey will require oestrogen therapy to initiate puberty, and will require oestrogen supplementation throughout the adult years. Most girls are also prescribed growth hormone therapy during childhood to enhance their growth. In adult years, patients with Turner's syndrome have combined endocrine and cardiology follow-up to monitor their hormonal treatment and cardiovascular problems, particularly aortic valve disease, coarctation and hypertension.
See Chapter 16 for further details.

Case 2: Constipation

1 Billy is constipated and his rectal bleeding in all likelihood is due to an anal fissure. The diagnosis of constipation is made on the basis of infrequent hard stools passed with difficulty. It should not be made on infrequent bowel movements alone.

2 Billy needs laxatives for a period to soften his stools and to allow the anal fissure to heal. The medication of choice is an iso-osmotic agent, polyethylene glycol (e.g. Movicol), although an osmotic laxative (lactulose) or a bowel stimulant is sometimes also used. Dietary advice is important—eating high-fibre foods such as wholewheat products and vegetables will help resolve the problem and prevent recurrence. Fruit and orange juice helps to soften stools. It is important that Billy has a good fluid intake.

The duration of treatment depends on how long he has been suffering from constipation and laxatives may be required for some months. Parents are often concerned about dependence on laxatives but this is not a problem in childhood.

3 You should consider Hirschsprung's if a child has delayed passage of meconium beyond the first 24 hours in the neonatal period, constipation from infancy and if there is significant weight faltering and poor growth.

4 Billy's soiling is no doubt due to overflow of liquid stool around constipated faeces. Good doses of laxative are required to clear the constipation; this can make the soiling worse in the short run.

5 Soiling is defined as the involuntary passage of faeces and results from leakage of liquid stool around impacted faeces. Encopresis is the *voluntary* passage of stools in inappropriate places (including underwear) by a child who is mature enough to be continent. It is indicative of severe behaviour problems.

6 Billy's prognosis is good provided laxatives are taken on a regular basis for some months and his diet contains good amounts of fibre to prevent constipation developing again.

Case 3: Cough and fever

1 You need to look for signs of respiratory distress. In childhood the signs are alar flaring, tachypnoea, tracheal tug and subcostal and intercostal retractions. If present they indicate significant respiratory distress.

2 In childhood it is very easy to hear transmitted noises from the upper respiratory tract. It can be difficult to differentiate these sounds from lower respiratory tract signs, which is why the external signs of respiratory distress are so important. The location of signs can also be unreliable.

3 If Jenny is poorly and showing signs of respiratory distress, a full blood count and blood culture are indicated along with a chest radiograph. If she seems well, once she is apyrexial, and there is no evidence of respiratory distress, she is unlikely to have serious lower respiratory tract disease and investigations are not required.

4 Given that the consolidation is focal rather than diffuse, a bacterial rather than viral cause is likely. Common organisms include *Streptococcus pneumoniae* and *Haemophilus influenzae* type B are most common. Less common are mycoplasma, group A streptococcus, and *Staphylococcus aureus*.

Case 4: Fits, faints and funny spells

1 The most likely diagnosis is breath-holding spells. Epilepsy and reflex anoxic seizures should also be considered in the differential diagnosis.

2 Breath-holding spells are characteristically precipitated by crying because of pain or temper. The child takes a deep breath, stops breathing, becomes deeply cyanotic and the limbs extend. Loss of consciousness does not usually occur, but if it does the child recovers rapidly with no postictal signs. Other types of fits, faints and funny spells do not usually have a precipitating event. Pallid (reflexic anoxic) spells can be confused with breath-holding spells, but differ in that they are caused by triggering of the vagal reflex following minor injury.

3 Always make sure that you get a description by someone who has observed the event. It can be helpful to ask the family to video an episode.

4 Reassurance is required. Parents can become quite terrified of these episodes and as a result may have difficulty in imposing discipline on the child for fear of provoking an attack.

5 These attacks are always benign and resolve before the child reaches school age.

Case 5: A jaundiced baby

1 This is early-onset jaundice (<24 h) and is therefore pathological and has to be taken seriously. You need to establish whether there are any risk factors for infection such as prolonged rupture of membranes or known maternal infection (high CRP, positive urine or HVS culture). It is also important to know the mother's blood group as this may be haemolytic disease of the newborn.

2 You should take blood to measure the serum bilirubin level and the babies blood group. A direct Coomb's test will establish whether there is maternal IgG antibody attached to the baby's red blood cells. A full blood count may show signs of anaemia and haemolysis and may show a leucocytosis if there is infection. CRP and blood culture should be performed.

3 The bilirubin result should be plotted on a graph (NICE treatment threshold graphs for term babies) against the time the sample was taken, in this case 12 hours of age. This shows that the bilirubin is well above the treatment line and on the exchange transfusion line.

4 As the bilirubin is 200 μmol/L at 12 h it is mandatory to start aggressive phototherapy with a high-luminescence device. The baby should be nursed naked (in an incubator if necessary) and with an open nappy to expose as much skin as possible to the light. A 'biliblanket' can be used to treat the underside of the baby simultaneously.

5 Serious consideration should be given to performing an exchange transfusion. This is particularly likely to be required if the Coomb's test is strongly positive, the newborn is already anaemic (due to in-utero haemolysis) or the bilirubin is rising rapidly (>8.5 μmol/L per hour). The transfusion lab should be alerted to prepare blood urgently. You may consider giving intravenous immunoglobulin to block antibody binding sites and slow the rate of haemolysis, while preparing for an exchange transfusion.

6 This child needs a formal BSER hearing test (due to the high peak bilirubin which is ototoxic) and should also be assessed for anaemia, since ongoing haemolysis can continue despite the jaundice resolving. This can lead to significant anaemia in the first 6 weeks of life. Folic acid supplements will help with erythropoesis.

Case 6: A baby with suspected cyanosis

1 It is important to establish whether this is central cyanosis by looking at the lips and tongue. If there is central cyanosis it is important to perform an urgent and thorough cardiac and respiratory examination. In the absence of any respiratory distress the cause is likely to be cardiac, especially if a murmur or abnormal pulses are present.

2 Oxygen saturation should be measured in the right arm and one of the feet. If both are <95% and there is no respiratory distress, or if there is a big drop between pre- and postductal saturation then CHD is likely. The fact that the baby has been breast-feeding well

makes persistent pulmonary hypertension of the newborn (PPHN) less likely. Chest radiograph may show an unusual heart shape or oligaemic lung fields but the saturation test is quicker and more useful.

3 If there are convincing signs of cyanotic CHD then the child should be admitted to the NICU urgently. Oxygen therapy is unlikely to be of benefit but is usually tried until the diagnosis is clear. Prostaglandin infusion should be commenced to keep the duct open and allow blood to cross the duct. A CXR and ECG may be useful, but the diagnostic test is an echocardiogram (cardiac ultrasound).

4 Yes. Polycythaemia can lead to a proportion of the haemoglobin being desaturated (without oxygen bound to it), making cyanosis more apparent, even in the absence of hypoxia. Polycythaemia is associated with poorly controlled maternal diabetes.

5 There is a wide variety of lesions that could be causing this picture, including pulmonary atresia, transposition of the great arteries and tricuspid atresia. TGA is 20 times more common in infants of diabetic mothers than in the background population. For the child to have been breast-feeding well it is likely that there was an ASD or VSD in addition, which allowed a degree of mixing of oxygenated blood within the heart. As the duct closed at 24 hours the baby would have become more cyanosed and more acidotic, due to tissue hypoxia.

Case 7: A swelling in the groin

1 Hydrocele, inguinal hernia, testicular torsion, trauma to the testes

2
• A hydrocele will transilluminate light from a pen-torch or otoscope, due to the presence of fluid around the testes. It is unusual for a hydrocele to recur having resolved in early childhood.
• -An inguinal hernia will become more prominent on coughing and it is difficult to delineate the upper margin of the swelling. It is not normally painful unless incarcerated.
• -Testicular torsion tends to occur in teenage boys and is acutely painful with a red tender mass present in the scrotum.
• Trauma may be caused by a direct blow to the scrotum, although there would normally be a clear history of this.
• Mumps is a viral infection that is now rare due to the MMR (mumps, measles, rubella) vaccine. It presents with malaise, fever and parotid swelling. It can be associated with orchitis (testicular inflammation) and can lead to subfertility.

3 These are the features of an incarcerated inguinal hernia. The fact that you cannot get above the swelling is because the hernial sac (usually containing bowel) is coming down the inguinal canal. If there is doubt an ultrasound can be helpful. The treatment is surgical reduction, with closure of the internal ring of the inguinal canal.

4 The danger of delayed treatment is if the incarcerated (irreducible) hernia contains bowel which is strangulated and becomes ischaemic. This can lead to necrosis or perforation of that segment of bowel, requiring resection and anastomosis.

Case 8: A collapsed child

1 You should follow the ABC approach. Shout for help and ask one of the children to get help. Check it is safe to approach (i.e. stop traffic if he is in the road) and establish whether he has an open airway. If he is still coughing then try to encourage effective coughs. It may be appropriate to try the Heimlich manoeuvre and alternate 5 abdominal thrusts with 5 back blows.

2 You need to get an urgent history from his friends as to what happened. This could be choking from an inhaled peanut or could possibly be severe anaphylaxis to peanuts. The latter would be more likely if there was a rash or swollen lips (angio-oedema) and wheeze or a known history (check for Medic-Alert bracelet). The former is more likely in this case with a history of choking and coughing. One of the boys admits they were throwing peanuts up in the air and trying to catch them in their mouths.

As he is now unconscious you need to open his airway ('sniffing the morning air' position) and check for breathing. If he is not breathing try to administer 5 rescue breaths by mouth to mouth, while pinching his nose. You should start CPR to try to dislodge the obstruction.

3 Once he is breathing he should be put in the recovery position until he regains consciousness. He needs to be taken to hospital urgently by ambulance.

4 A chest radiograph may be indicated to check for signs of aspiration and to exclude a foreign body still being lodged in his lower airway. If there are signs of persistent lobar or lung collapse a bronchoscopy may be needed to retrieve any further foreign body from his lower airway.

Case 9: A child with vomiting and altered conscious level

1 Yes. Altered conscious level is potentially life threatening as impaired consciousness means that the airway can be compromised. If a partially conscious patient vomits they may aspirate and risk respiratory arrest. Intervention to protect the airway includes positioning of the neck and chin and consider whether nasogastric tube should be placed to aspirate stomach contents. Call anaesthetist as airway intubation may be needed.

2 Glasgow Coma Score (GCS) total 9:
• Eye opening 3 (to verbal command)
• Movement 4 (flexion with pain)
• Speech 2 (incomprehensible sounds)

3 He needs high-dependency one-to-one monitoring to observe for any further deterioration which would require urgent resuscitation. He should be moved to a resuscitation room or high-dependency unit. Continuous physiological monitoring of oxygen saturation, ECG, pulse rate, is necessary. High-frequency measurement of blood pressure, pupil responses, GCS, temperature and fluid balance is needed.

4 Diabetic ketoacidosis is suggested by the pattern of breathing, which indicates metabolic acidosis, and the history of nocturnal enuresis.

5 Blood glucose, gas, ketones will confirm diabetic ketoacidosis: pH < 7.3, bicarbonate < 15, blood glucose > 11 mmol/L. Blood urea and electrolytes will help guide fluid management.

6
• Intensive monitoring during correction of metabolic and fluid derangement with aim to restore pH, glucose, potassium and fluid balance.
• Intravenous insulin is started 1 hour after intravenous fluids to stop ketogenesis and gradually correct blood glucose.
• Monitor particularly for cerebral oedema which can present with bradycardia or headache.

Case 10: A 3-month-old baby with bruises

1 A detailed family health and social history is needed to understand the baby's pattern of care, who has been involved, the family's background, whether there are any other children and whether there have been any previous child protection issues. It is important to ask about risk factors for child abuse such as domestic violence and substance abuse. It is important to ask whether there is any family history of bleeding disorders such as Von Willebrand's disease or other indicators of familial bleeding tendencies such as maternal heavy menstrual bleeding.

2 Baby's general health, weight gain, head circumference, conscious level. Any signs of injuries in hidden areas such as the frenulum of the tongue. Any sign of bone pain when the baby is handled. Any other soft tissue injury signs. Fundoscopy to look for retinal haemorrhages

3 Blood count and clotting to exclude thrombocytopenia or coagulation disorder. Ophthalmology review to examine for retinal haemorrhages. Skeletal survey to check for any recent or old bone fractures. Brain imaging should be considered to check for any subdural bleeding. The bruises should be photographed.

4 If signs of possible inflicted (non-accidental) injury are present then the case must be jointly managed with local authority social work professionals and police to investigate the presentation and agree a plan for the future safeguarding of the child before discharge from hospital.

Case 11: A 14-year-old girl with cystic fibrosis

1
• Growth and weight gain are closely linked to respiratory function. At age 14 she should be progressing through puberty and this is also a sign of good control.
• Lung function test (spirometry) results.
• Sputum culture, particularly any more aggressive chronic respiratory infection organisms such as pseudomonas.
• Chest radiograph changes.
• Annual screening tests of vitamin levels, liver function, glucose tolerance test.

2 Transition to adulthood is a complex process of increasing independence from parents, self-reliance and change in lifestyle. The focus of the consultation moves from discussion with parents and child to more direct discussion with the young person. It is helpful for paediatric and adult clinical teams to work together to achieve gradual transition and continuity of care.

Specific health issues: ongoing surveillance of respiratory function, respiratory infection, maintaining nutrition and weight. Young adult lifestyle advice relating to contraception and fertility, smoking, drug and alcohol use. Cystic fibrosis related diabetes and liver disease become more common with increasing age.

Case 12: A 12-year-old girl with progressive tiredness

1 The history is suggestive of chronic fatigue syndrome, which is debilitating fatigue of long duration in which routine investigations have failed to identify any other pathological cause. Other causes of this sort of presentation include:
• Haematology/oncology—anaemia, leukaemia, lymphoma
• Autoimmune—systemic lupus erythematosus, dermatomyositis
• Infection—tuberculosis, hepatitis, Epstein–Barr virus

• Drug-related—substance abuse, excessive anti-epileptic medication
• Endocrine—diabetes, Addison's, hypothyroid
• Gastrointestinal—coeliac disease, inflammatory bowel disease
• Psychiatric—depression, eating disorder

2 Detailed history of the family and school background is important. Is there a history of illness affecting a close relative? What are the family and child's beliefs about the illness mechanism and approach to management?

3 Full blood count and film, ESR, CRP, blood glucose, blood biochemistry, creatinine kinase, thyroid function, viral antibody titres to Epstein–Barr virus. Urine analysis for blood, protein, infection.

These are the initial screening investigations. Other investigations may be indicated if there are specific features in the history or examination.

4 The following steps are helpful in managing chronic fatigue:

• If possible the process of investigation should be concluded quickly and alternative diagnoses excluded.
• The diagnosis should be communicated carefully so that child and family understand what is known about the condition and the uncertainty about the aetiology. It is helpful to explain that this is a pattern of illness that is not well understood but is seen repeatedly in a large number of young people and adults.
• A combined approach of work with a team including paediatrician, physiotherapist and mental health staff is helpful to address the physical and psychological issues together. Gradual 'pacing' of activity and exercise to build up tolerance is recommended. Psychological support to help understand any background problems and cope with the social withdrawal and anxiety related to the illness is often helpful. Work with school to enable progressive staged re-inclusion alongside physical rehabilitation. In some situations specialist pain team advice can be helpful.

Index